A Nurse's Guide to Presenting and Publishing

Dare to Share

Kathleen T. Heinrich, PhD, RN

Principal, KTH Consulting
Guilford, Connecticut

JONES AND BARTLETT PUBLISHERS

Sudbury, Massachusetts

BOSTON   TORONTO   LONDON   SINGAPORE

World Headquarters

Jones and Bartlett Publishers
40 Tall Pine Drive
Sudbury, MA 01776
978-443-5000
info@jbpub.com
www.jbpub.com

Jones and Bartlett Publishers
Canada
6339 Ormindale Way
Mississauga, Ontario L5V 1J2
Canada

Jones and Bartlett Publishers
International
Barb House, Barb Mews
London W6 7PA
United Kingdom

Jones and Bartlett's books and products are available through most bookstores and online book-sellers. To contact Jones and Bartlett Publishers directly, call 800-832-0034, fax 978-443-8000, or visit our website www.jbpub.com.

Substantial discounts on bulk quantities of Jones and Bartlett's publications are available to corporations, professional associations, and other qualified organizations. For details and specific discount information, contact the special sales department at Jones and Bartlett via the above contact information or send an email to specialsales@jbpub.com.

The authors, editor, and publisher have made every effort to provide accurate information. However, they are not responsible for errors, omissions, or for any outcomes related to the use of the contents of this book and take no responsibility for the use of the products and procedures described. Treatments and side effects described in this book may not be applicable to all people; likewise, some people may require a dose or experience a side effect that is not described herein. Drugs and medical devices are discussed that may have limited availability controlled by the Food and Drug Administration (FDA) for use only in a research study or clinical trial. Research, clinical practice, and government regulations often change the accepted standard in this field. When consideration is being given to use of any drug in the clinical setting, the healthcare provider or reader is responsible for determining FDA status of the drug, reading the package insert, and reviewing prescribing information for the most up-to-date recommendations on dose, precautions, and contraindications, and determining the appropriate usage for the product. This is especially important in the case of drugs that are new or seldom used.

Production Credits

Executive Editor: Kevin Sullivan
Acquisitions Editor: Emily Ekle
Associate Editor: Amy Sibley
Editorial Assistant: Patricia Donnelly
Production Director: Amy Rose
Associate Production Editor: Wendy Swanson
Associate Marketing Manager: Rebecca Wasley
Manufacturing and Inventory Control
  Supervisor: Amy Bacus
Cover Design: Kristin E. Ohlin
Text Design: Arlene Apone
Composition: Arlene Apone
Printing and Binding: Malloy, Inc.
Cover Printing: Malloy, Inc.

Library of Congress Cataloging-in-Publication Data
Heinrich, Kathleen T.
  A nurse's guide to presenting and publishing : dare to share / Kathleen. T. Heinrich.
    p. ; cm.
  Includes bibliographical references and index.
  ISBN-13: 978-0-7637-4679-7 (pbk. : alk. paper)
  ISBN-10: 0-7637-4679-7 (pbk. : alk. paper) 1. Nursing—Authorship 2. Nursing literature—Marketing. 3. Public speaking. 4. Creative ability.
  [DNLM: 1. Creativeness—Nurses' Instruction. 2. Nurse's Role. 3. Nurses—psychology. 4. Publishing—Nurses' Instruction. 5. Writing—Nurses' Instruction. BF 408 H469n 2008] I. Title.
  RT24.H47 2008
  610.73—dc22
                        2007026917

6048

Printed in the United States of America
11 10 09 08 07 10 9 8 7 6 5 4 3 2 1

Dedication

This book is dedicated to the students and faculty colleagues at Yale University, the University of San Diego, and the University of Hartford who enticed me into teaching nurses how to present and write for publication.

Contents

Section 3: Small Steps to Write About What You Do

Section 4: Small Steps to Cultivate Support Circles

Section 5: Small Steps: Send Off

About the Author

Kathleen T. Heinrich, PhD, RN is a popular speaker, prolific author, nationally recognized educational researcher, and award winning educator. After receiving a master's degree in community mental health nursing in 1976, Kathleen's yearning to learn would take her to Big Sur, California to study Gestalt Therapy and to Kusnacht, Switzerland to study Jungian psychology. Balancing a psychotherapy practice with a faculty position, she received a doctoral degree in higher education with a special-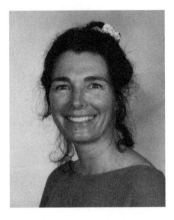
ization in the adult learner in 1988. When Kathleen's research suggested that nurses need to be systematically prepared to present and publish, she crisscrossed the country attending creative writing conferences to learn how to do just that. Melding her background in Jungian psychology with her educational expertise, Kathleen developed an integrative approach that gives nurses the self-confidence and the know-how to take the dare to share. After 25 years of teaching in RN-BSN, master's, and doctoral programs at three universities, Kathleen resigned her tenured professorship in 2004 to open KTH Consulting. She now shares her evidence-based, best presenting and publishing practices with nursing groups in colleges, universities, and healthcare agencies as a way for them to enhance their careers, recover their passion for the profession, and foster zestful workplaces.

Contributors

Contributing Authors

Cynthia Clark, RN, PhD
Professor
Department of Nursing
Boise State University
Boise, ID

Kelley Connor, RNC, MSN
Instructor
Department of Nursing
College of Health Science
Boise State University
Boise, ID

Melissa Dayton, MM, MA
Adult Educator
Capitol Region Education Council
Hartford, CT

Molly Davison-Price, RN, MSN
Clinical Nurse II
University of Connecticut
    Health Center
Farmington, CT

Laurel Halloran, PhD, APRN
Professor of Nursing
Department of Nursing
Western Connecticut State University
Nurse Practitioner
Pulmonary Department
Danbury Hospital
Danbury, CT

**Susan Luparell, PhD, APRN,
    BC, CNE**
Assistant Professor
College of Nursing
Montana State University
Great Falls, MT

Irene O'Day, RN (retired)
Program Presenter, Integrative
    Medicine Modalities
Associate of the Sisters of Mercy
    Northeast
Prison Volunteer–Peace Activist
Clinton, CT

Diana King Mixon, RN, MSN
Associate Professor
Department of Nursing
College of Health Science
Boise State University
Boise, ID

Christina Purpora, MSN, RN, CCRN
Doctoral Student
School of Nursing
University of California
San Francisco, CA

Beverly Sastri, MBA
Speaker, Consultant on Living
  Your Fullest Potential
Originator, *Live Like You Mean It!*
  Workshops
Power Source Now, LLC
Guilford, CT

Pam G. Walker, RN, MSN
Assistant Professor of Nursing
Goodwin College
East Hartford, CT

Other Contributors

Kevin T. Besse, RN, MSN
Instructor
Department of Nursing
College of Nursing and Allied
  Health Professions
University of Louisiana at Lafayette
Lafayette, LA

Joan C. Borgatti, RN, MEd
Author/Editor/Writing Coach
Borgatti Communications
Former Editorial Director,
  Nursing Spectrum
Natick, MA

Susan Brinigar, RN, LMT
Kripalu Yoga Teacher
Guilford, CT

Peggy L. Chinn, RN, PhD, FAAN
Editor, *Advances in Nursing Science*
Professor Emerita
School of Nursing
University of Connecticut
Storrs, CT

Suzanne Hall Johnson, RN, MN, CNS
Editor Emeritus, *Dimensions of
  Critical Care Nursing*
Editor Emeritus, *Nurse Author
  & Editor*
Lakewood, CO

Louise C. Marks, ACSW
Storyteller & Writer, Seeker
  & Sailor
Westbrook, CT

James E. Mattson
Editor, *Reflections on Nursing
  Leadership (RNL)*
Honor Society of Nursing, Sigma
  Theta Tau International
Indianapolis, IN

Lisa Nowak, RN, MSN
Editor, *ASNC Newsletter*
Nursing Supervisor
West Hartford Public Schools
West Hartford, CT

Melinda Granger Oberleitner, RN, DNS, APRN, CNS
Review Editor & Former Associate
 Editor, *Oncology Nursing Forum*
Professor and Department Head
Associate to the Dean
College of Nursing and Allied
 Health Professions
University of Louisiana at Lafayette
Lafayette, LA

Marilyn H. Oermann, RN, PhD, FAAN
Editor, *Journal of Nursing Care Quality*
Professor and Chair, Adult and
 Geriatric Health Division
School of Nursing
The University of North Carolina
 at Chapel Hill
Chapel Hill, NC

Karen A. Owen, RN, MSN
School Nurse
W. C. Polson Middle School
Madison, CT

Sue Preneta
Dancer, Choreographer, Teacher
Art Acquisitions Consultant
Freelance Editor, Designer,
 and Producer
Guilford, CT

Kelly Rossler, RN, MSN
Instructor
Department of Nursing
College of Nursing and Allied
 Health Professions
University of Louisiana at Lafayette
Lafayette, LA

Suzanne P. Smith, RN, EdD, FAAN
Editor-in-Chief, *The Journal of Nursing Administration* and *Nurse Educator*
Bradenton, FL

Prelude

Tell your stories. As nurses, we hear this all the time. So why don't we? Especially when other disciplines see presenting and publishing as acts of professional generosity and a shared responsibility. My guess is that it's the mixed messages. Tell your stories, *but* don't stand out, don't call attention to yourself. Don't talk too much about what you do or you'll be seen as selfish in a caring profession. It makes me realize just how daring nurses must be to share who they are and what they do.

There's no question that silence used to protect us. After all, for over 300 years healers in Europe were called witches and burned at the stake. When keeping quiet meant staying alive, we learned to silence ourselves. Now our silence is holding us back. There are those inside and outside of nursing who are rooting for us to speak our truth—visionaries such as Bernice Buresh and Suzanne Gordon who wrote the book *From Silence to Voice* because they believe that our survival as a profession depends on sharing our stories.

As a teacher and a writer, I know that sharing begets sharing, which, in turn, leads to insights that transform the way we see ourselves and practice nursing. Because storytelling is the essence of presenting and publishing, *Dare to Share* is full of stories and invitations to share yours. Then, beyond the joy of self-expression, your sharings will enrich our cache of oral and written stories that inform present practice and ensure our future by creating a legacy to build upon.

Reader's Quiz

Is *Dare to Share* the Book for You?

Circle the following items that best describe you:

- I am a nurse.
- I believe that what I do is important.
- I am passionate about what I do.
- I'd like to share what I do by presenting.
- I'd like to share what I do by publishing.
- I have to share what I do to keep my job.
- I want the exuberant, glitter-in-the-eye that nurses have who dare to share.
- I wish I had a wise and knowledgeable mentor to help me share what I do.
- I yearn for a circle of colleagues who dare to share what they do.
- I yearn for a circle of colleagues who dare me to share what I do.
- I'd like to help nurse colleagues share what they do.
- I'm intimidated by the idea of sharing what I do.

Ironically, it's public speaking and writing—the very activities that nurses fear the most—that can kindle or rekindle nurses' passion for nursing. If you circled two or more of the quiz items, turn intimidation into intrigue as you follow the small steps set out in this guidebook—shift your perspective, reflect on yourself as a presenter and/or author, practice strategies and skills, and form support circles. Then, whether you're a student, a staff nurse, an advanced practice nurse, or an educator, administrator, or entrepreneur, you'll know how to transform your practice into presentations and publications. To find out more, turn the page.

Preface: Why I Wrote This Guidebook

I am a part of all that I have met.

Alfred Lord Tennyson

As a nurse, you find ways to help people in circumstances that call out their best and their worst every single day. Even though you may not say it aloud, this is your unique contribution to nursing. Somewhere along the way you may have gotten the impression that it's selfish to share your "something special" publicly. This is a mistaken belief. Far from being conceited or boastful, sharing what you do is a great way to give back. Think of it this way. When you keep your special something to yourself, only you, the people whose lives you touch, and a few colleagues know what you do, whereas a single presentation or article can reach more people than a lifetime of practice.

With all your experiences as a nurse, you're halfway to sharing what you do. *Dare to Share* takes you the rest of the way by showing you how. What you may not realize is how energizing it is to present and publish. Not only will your passion for nursing be ignited, sharing what you do can change your life. You'll delight in dialogues that deepen your ideas and spark insights in others. Your e-mail in-box will fill with messages from colleague–friends across the country and the world who mentor you from afar. As opportunities you never dreamed possible come your way, you'll jump out of bed eager to start the day.

All this can happen to you. Why am I so sure? Because it's happening to me. You may be thinking, sure, that's easy to say when you know how to share what you do. Actually, it's just the opposite. My dare came from not knowing how, and, as you'll see, taking that dare has been turning obstacles into challenges and colleagues into allies ever since.

My Call to Adventure

My initiation started with a flop. After I graduated from my master's program in 1976, I worked in a day hospital as a psychiatric clinical specialist. When our team talked about publishing an article about our treatment approach, I volunteered to write the first draft. After all, how hard could it be? I'd gotten "A"s in English all through school; as a college freshman, my English teacher encouraged me to consider writing if ever I tired of nursing. When I tried to draft our article, I had no idea where to begin, what journal might want it, or how to contact an editor. Finally, overwhelmed and frustrated, I gave up. Who knew that this misadventure would ignite my desire to share what I do?

Allies Intervene

Several years after this aborted attempt and in my second year of teaching, I attended Suzanne Hall Johnson's writing workshop in 1979. After 2 days of learning her step-by-step approach, I knew how to turn an idea into an article. It would be 5 years before I used Suzanne's steps to craft a letter querying another Suzanne—Suzanne Smith, the editor of *Nurse Educator (NE)*—about her interest in an idea I had for an article. Elated by *NE* editor Suzanne's positive response, I submitted my manuscript (this is what you call an article before it's published). When it was rejected, despair turned to relief when Suzanne Smith helped me to revise it. Seeing my name in print the first time was such a high that, as Suzanne Hall Johnson predicted, writing articles became an addictive pleasure. I am grateful to both Suzannes for initiating me into the technical side of publishing and for mentoring me to this day.

Weaving Together My Clinical Specialty and Teaching

In the early 1980s, I awoke every morning grateful for my life. I was renting a cottage overlooking Long Island Sound, and my work life balanced teaching full-time on a nursing faculty with practicing as a part-time nurse-therapist. This equilibrium was upset by an ultimatum from my university—either enroll in a doctoral program or no more teaching contracts. My desire to teach won out, and I ended up in a doctoral program in 1984. Having taught nurses for 10 years, I reveled in the coursework that revolved around adult learning. My fear of statistics, on the other hand, gave the term "math anxiety" a new meaning. I sobbed for 3 hours after my first quantitative (a.k.a. numbers) research class. Unless I could get someone else to do my research for me, how was I going to write a dissertation?

A solution emerged when a professor named Dr. Linda Lewis noticed my ability to organize people's stories into themes. She encouraged me to consider a qualitative dissertation in which stories, not numbers, are the data. With Linda at the helm of my dissertation committee, I interviewed 18 women graduates from a doctoral program in education about their relationships with male and female advisors. I have Linda to thank for showing me how to translate a talent honed as a psychotherapist into the dissertation research project that earned me a doctorate.

My Initiation of Small Steps Continues

After graduating from my doctoral program in December 1989, I felt like Rip Van Winkle awakening after 4 years to find that my dream faculty position had become a nightmare. Eight months later I resigned, said good-bye to my therapy clients, and headed west for a new faculty position. Betwixt and between identities, I was no longer a nurse-therapist and not yet a nurse-scholar. Within the first week of starting my new job, I was told that I needed a "program of research" to teach in the doctoral program. Not even sure what a program of research was, I flailed around for a topic. When I learned that the first cohort of nurses was graduating from the doctoral program, I knew I'd found the participants for my next study. A faculty grant funded my interviewing graduates once a year for the next 5 years. Since I'd graduated only a year before these 16 women, we were all new-docs. Little wonder that their issues were my issues. Even though we were all committed to becoming scholars, less than a handful had mentors. The rest of us suffered from "mentor-hunger"—a deep yearning for a wise mentor to introduce us to the world of nurse scholars and researchers. By the end of the fifth year, we were comfortable with being called "doctor" and on a high from flexing our scholarly muscles by presenting and publishing. While awaiting those mentors who never materialized, we'd created support circles of colleagues who mentored us. These support circles confirmed what I'd long suspected—becoming a scholar is a relational process that unfolds over time.

Would a Support Circle of Colleague-Mentors Help Doctoral Students Become Scholars?

I thought it was just me who felt *less* confident about myself after graduation than when I entered my doctoral program until I discovered that many of my 16 study participants, along with 200 women new-docs in education participating in Debra Sikes's (1996) study, said they felt the same way. What could I do to prevent this from happening to other women? As a student of Carl Jung's school of psychology, I knew the power of myth to give meaning to human dilemmas. So when I came across an article by Kathleen Noble[1] that applied the metaphor of the hero's journey to women's lives, I wondered if reframing doctoral study as a heroic passage would help a group of women doctoral students to become scholars without losing themselves in the process.

Intertwining psychology with education, the study "Doctoral Study as Heroic Journey" was designed to answer this question. Ten doctoral students, women between the ages of 38 to 55, volunteered for a weekend retreat. In the process of reflecting on their lives through journal writing and artwork, they reclaimed personal voices shaken by mid-life challenges (e.g., empty nests, divorces, searches for a more meaningful career path, etc.). Sharing their experiences freed participants to open themselves to the challenges of doctoral study. Meeting only one afternoon a semester over the next 18 months, this group of caring women became a circle of scholarly caring. As participants' personal voices matured into scholarly voices, reflection became action. Our support circle gave some the courage to become passionate scholars by pursuing dissertation topics dear to their hearts regardless of the political risks. In the process, they taught me that becoming a passionate scholar is a heroic journey in which self-reflection plays as much a part as technical strategies and relational skills.

Paying It Forward

By 1994, I'd watched too many doctoral students struggle with scholarly writing. It was no surprise that, after years of quoting experts' opinions, even doctoral candidates completing dissertations were hard pressed to articulate their own viewpoints. From doctoral students to new docs, many had trouble translating their school papers into presentations or publications. Could sharing what I'd learned about writing from the two Suzannes help? To find out, just before resigning my West Coast faculty post, I piloted a "Writing for Publication" workshop for doctoral students. Borrowing from my psychology background, we first discussed how the voices of "inner critics" complicate our writing process. Then we dug into the technical details. After a day filled with views of the Pacific Ocean, whoops of laughter, and great food, doctoral-student participants came away with a newfound confidence in their ability to translate ideas into query letters and publishable products. These women confirmed that a psychological–educational–relational approach made scholarly writing doable and fun.

"You Don't Know How to Write in a Scholarly Way"

These words popped out of my mouth as I wrangled with a group of master's students over three-page papers that were unreadable. Having moved back East, I was an adjunct professor teaching an introductory theory course. Beneath my exasperation, I was scared. Sure, I presented and published regularly. That West Coast, "Writing for Publication" workshop proved that I could teach doctoral students who already knew how to write like scholars to publish. Now I needed to learn how to help master's students convert scholarly writing into the publishable products they needed to graduate. But who would teach me? As I wondered what my college English teacher was doing these days, an answer came clear—creative writers. With neither the time nor the money for a graduate program in creative writing, I continued my own education by subscribing to *Poets & Writers: From Inspiration to Publication (P & W)*. Using the *P & W* conference listings as a guide, I began traveling to writing retreats in knock-out locations from Connecticut to California. In between, I attended authors' book readings at our local, independent bookstore. Every time I learned something applicable, I'd add it to the "Writing for

Publication" workshop. Without those unreadable student papers, I might never have taken the dare to learn to teach students to write.

Angry Students Become Allies

When I became the coordinator of a graduate program preparing nurse educators in 1998, I imagined myself encircled by adoring students. Instead, I encountered the angriest bunch I'd met in 20 years of teaching. The first night of class, they announced there were 210 days until graduation and things went downhill from there. By mid-year, I'd found a way to turn sour into sweet. During our accreditation visit the year before, the National League for Nursing (NLN) visitors said we needed a program assessment process that folded student evaluation feedback into curriculum design. Since we had no idea how to do this, my faculty colleagues were only too happy to give the go-ahead when I suggested that the angry students help us evaluate our program.

University funding allowed me to train master's student volunteers to conduct focus groups with the 68 angry graduates. When asked what it had been like being a student in this program, graduates' responses revealed that beneath their anger, they were scared. Here they were graduating not knowing how to conduct research or translate findings into publishable products. Their recommendation? "If you want to graduate students who know how to publish, you need to prepare students to write for publication." Without the NLN visitors' mandate, we would have bid a grateful adieu to this angry group, never asking them what would improve our curriculum.

The "Perspective Transformation" Course Prepares Students as Scholars

To meet the angry students' recommendations, three graduate-student partners and I wrote an NLN 2001 grant to fund the design, teaching, and evaluation of a course to prepare master's students as scholars. We defined nurse-scholars as those who articulate ideas, verbally and in writing, that are grounded in the literature. Adapting what I'd learned from my research with doctoral women scholars, the first third of the course developed students' reflection skills, the second third refined their technical strategies, and the last third enhanced their relational skills. Final evaluations confirmed that students left this course confident that they had the requisite scholarly skill set and the faculty support to complete the program. This evidence-based course, "Perspective Transformation: Socialization into a Community of Scholarly Caring" now introduces entering RN-BSNs and graduate students to an entire curriculum that prepares them to present and publish after graduation. For this, we have those angry students to thank.

Faculty Members Feel Like Scholar-Imposters, Too

During the 5 years I was learning to help students share what they do, I headed up a university committee that assessed what helped and hindered faculty from turning their teaching into scholarship. Although knowledgeable in their subjects, we discovered that most professors on our campus had neither been taught to teach nor mentored as teacher-scholars. So we designed a six-session, university-wide, faculty development workshop series called "Work Smart: Turn Your Teaching into Scholarship."

Just as with students, developing faculty participants' ability to self-reflect, use technical strategies and skills, and create support circles helped them to present and publish. Whether artists or engineers, musicians or chemists, political scientists or nurses, intense dialogue and inspired suggestions from colleagues transformed these educators' trepidation to exuberance. Without knowing it, helping students and faculty colleagues to turn their teaching into projects, proposals, presentations, and publications was giving my life a whole new direction.

My Passion Becomes My Business

After 30 years, I finally had words to describe the "special something" that I bring to nursing. It's my psycho–educational–relational approach to presenting and publishing that informs and inspires nurses to dare to share what they do. Secure in this knowledge, I traded a steady paycheck for life as an entrepreneur when I resigned my tenured professorship in 2004. As the principal of my own company—KTH Consulting—I work with nursing groups in academic and practice settings who want to or are expected to share what they do.

This Book

The small steps shared in this book have helped hundreds of students, staff nurses, advanced practice nurses, nurse educators, managers, and entrepreneurs to take the dare to share what they do. Now you can learn to do the same. For the first time ever, these evidence-based steps are contained in one book. Meant as a portable mentor, this guidebook introduces you to all four steps: *shift in perspective* to see yourself as creative; *self-reflect* to explore your "inner landscape"; *strategies and skills* to practice the techniques and tools; and *support circles* to develop mindful relationships with colleague–friends.

Written for every nurse, *Dare to Share* can be used as a handbook by individuals or small groups in practice settings; as a textbook for baccalaureate, graduate, and doctoral students; or as a companion text for professional development, faculty development, or continuing education workshops. *Dare to Share* contains everything you need for a journey sure to make your eyes glitter, give new meaning to your life, and encircle you with various colleague–friends. The sooner you turn the page, the sooner you'll be ready to take the dare to share what you do.

Kathleen T. Heinrich
Tuttle's Point
Guilford, CT

Reference

1. Noble, K. D. (1990). The female hero: A quest for healing and wholeness. *Women and Therapy, 9*(4), 3–18.

Acknowledgments

As Felix Frankfurter once said, "Gratitude is the least articulate of feelings especially when it is deep." My gratitude is as wise as it is deep; if it weren't for my support circle, you wouldn't be reading these words because this book wouldn't exist. For this, I have my colleague–friends and resonators; creatives and playmates; wise ones and mentors; and friends and family to thank—most of whom, unless it says otherwise, are nurses.

Words cannot convey my gratefulness to those colleague–friends and resonators who call me to be true to my voice and to my work. A special thanks to Molly Davison-Price and Christina Purpora for peer editing the *Dare to Share* manuscript with a mix of honesty and affirmation that never failed to calm my raging impostor. To Katharine White, nurse turned life coach, for showing me how building personal foundations and support circles can make it safe to give up the security of a tenured position to write this book. To Beverly Sastri, visioning consultant, for teaching me to craft a vision for a new work life and guiding me to actualize that vision with trust and courage. To Cindy Clark and Susan Luparell for adding zest to my life as we celebrate each other's dares to share in our Cosmic Connection. To Dori Sullivan for supporting my dream of consulting from the first and for connecting me with Amy Sibley at Jones and Bartlett. To Dori's faculty group at Sacred Heart University, Joan Fisler and her Association of Women Business Leaders, and Melinda Oberleitner and her faculty group at the University of Louisiana at Lafayette for the opportunity to refine the presenting and publishing strategies shared in these pages.

Thanks to the creatives and playmates who teach me as much about life as they do about their craft. To Ronnie Ford and Lori Ruskin for reawakening my love of dance and movement. To Brendan Loughlin, my art teacher, for reigniting my childhood passion for painting flowers and skies like Van Gogh in sessions that interlaced laughter and life lessons with learning his Pastac method. To Sue Preneta, my dance teacher, for sharing her joyous music mixes and choreography as generously as her knowledge of publishing. To Susan Brinigar for refreshing my writing-weary mind with yoga postures and supplying the perfect quotation for *Dare to Share* chapters week after week. To Tess Morrison, intuitive visioner, for her humor and sage insights that helped me to see the larger meaning in writing this book. To my "Sagittarian Sisters," Madonna Boehlert and Ann Nye, for rescuing me from terminal serious-ity with their exuberance, love of beauty, and playfulness, and for conjuring up the garden party to celebrate the blossoming of this book.

Thanks to the wise ones and mentors who show me the way to mature into this third phase of life with grace and dignity. To my dearest "Goddesses on the Rocks," Mary Jo Barend, Sherry Hartwell, and Pam Culley-McCullough, for California reunions that helped me regain the perspective to write this book with compassion. To Irene O'Day for introducing me to the Namaste group that meets on-the-lake at Elmira Ingersoll and Mary Saylor Muhlhausen's Harmony House. To Elmira and Mary for being the wise women who, at 98 and 100, live the power of support circles by making all of us feel seen and appreciated. To Clovis and Grady, for sharing their enchanted place in Big Sur where I wrote parts of this book and for reminding me that living artfully is creating beauty in the everyday—fruit from the trees, vegetables from the garden, and good friends with whom to share the bounty. To Dorothy Cochrane, my yoga teacher, for her gift of appreciating the moment and for inspiring me to do the same.

Thanks to my friends and family who show me the power of unconditional love. To Melissa Dayton, for accompanying me every step of the way from reading awful first drafts to UPS-ing final copyedits to the publisher and for keeping me centered in mind and body with our long walks. To Frank and Mildred Scaglia, my grandparents, for teaching me that creativity flowers in gardens amidst strawberries, tomatoes, and stories well told. To Carl Otto Heinrich, my father, for bequeathing me the virtues of patience and perseverance and always being proud of what I accomplished in the world. I pray that he can see this book from the beyond. To Francis Scaglia Heinrich, my mother, for paving the way for future peer mentors by encouraging me to read, listening to my every speech, and typing all my school papers. To Ginny Tietjen, my virtual mother-in-law, for dinners shared at the Fish Tale and for asking, even when there wasn't much to tell, how the book was going. And, last and most of all, to Chris Tietjen, my loving partner, for his hanging in during the 22 years between writing my dissertation and this first book, always knowing whether I needed a kiss or a kick in the pants, a walk or a talk, and never shying away from giving what was needed most.

Introduction

Whatever you can do, or dream you can, begin it. Boldness has genius, power and magic in it.

Goethe

Are you and your colleagues feeling overwhelmed by increasing demands to present and publish? No wonder. With universities shifting the emphasis from teaching to scholarship and hospitals pursuing external recognition awards like Magnet Status, more and more nurses are expected to share what they do. Not only is professional nursing in the new millennium a call to presenting and publishing,[1] *all* nurses are expected to add to our knowledge base.[2]

The timing couldn't be worse! Just when overextended nurses fear a future of baby boomer retirements with too few nurse educators to prepare new recruits, they are being asked to do something they don't know how or don't have the time to do. Nurses often recoil from the dare to share because:

1. We are taught to practice nursing, we're not taught to present and publish.
2. Presenting and publishing are add-ons to heavy workloads.
3. There are too few mentors to go around.

Perhaps this explains why presenting and publishing remain the exclusive territory of a chosen few. Until now, the how-tos have been kept as secret as the formula for making Coca-Cola. To make it possible for *all* nurses to share, three things need to change:

1. Nurse educators must learn how to present and publish what they do.
2. Nursing students must be prepared to present and publish in their academic programs.
3. Nurses must learn to mentor each other before and after graduation.

When this happens, sharing will become a choice rather than an impossible dream for nurses, regardless of age, life stage, educational preparation, or specialty area.

What's in It for You to Read This Book?

Dare to Share begins where many nurses begin—by sharing what they do with professional audiences and readers. If you want to present in venues and/or publish in newsletters, magazines, and journals for nurse–generalists or specialists, *Dare to Share* demystifies the process. After reading this guidebook, you'll know how to find a slant that intrigues, the right audience, the best format, and a fitting venue or vehicle. Then it won't matter if your presentation is an inspirational speech for your hospital's Nurses' Day celebration or a paper delivered at a professional conference; or whether you're writing an article for a general nursing audience in *Nursing 2005* or for experts in your specialty in *Cardiac Care Nursing*. You'll be able to turn every project—clinical intervention, curricular innovation, or administrative strategy—into presentations and publications.

How to Get the Most Out of This Guidebook

It's just like physical exercise! To get the benefit from *Dare to Share,* you must participate. Beyond the desire, you'll need patience and persistence. If you're feeling hesitant about fitting one more thing into your overstuffed schedule, don't. Written for busy nurses like you, the chapters in this book are three to five pages short. You can finish most chapters in 15 minutes and walk away with an action plan for taking the next small step. Because chapters are short, there are a lot of them. The good news is that there are only four sections and four subsections. Should you lose track, check for the box in the upper right corner of the opening page of each chapter. The heading at the top left corner of this box tells you whether you're reading a chapter in the section devoted to *Small Steps, Present What You Do, Write About What You Do,* or *Support Circles*. The heading in the lower right corner of this box—*Shift In Perspective, Self-Reflect, Strategies and Skills, Support Circles*—describes the learning activity particular to the topic discussed in each chapter.

Rather than the formal, academic style of most nursing textbooks, *Dare to Share* reads like nurses speak in real life. Using simple language and everyday situations, ideas are clearly stated, easy to understand, and immediately applicable. Each chapter opens with a story or a quiz, highlights key points, and ends with an application exercise along with a tip that's a practical, punch-line summary. There are three different types of boxes—Information Boxes, Jot Boxes, and Worksheets. Information Boxes contain definitions of terms and related concepts, such as free-writes. Chapters also include blank Jot Boxes for your responses to learning activities. As you complete each Jot Box, you're teaching yourself another small step. Because I never ask you to do something I don't do, my responses to many of the activities are provided as examples. If reading my answers is helpful, great. If not, just ignore them. The same goes for the Worksheets that include quizzes and questionnaires for you to complete. Written in an informed-conversational style, you'll learn from the stories of students, colleagues, mentors, and tormentors, as well as insights drawn from the literature in nursing, psychology, education, and creative writing. In addition, I've asked the best presenters, authors, editors, peer mentors, peer editors, and partners I know to write "storytelling chapters" that give you the real scoop on what it's like to dare to share. Taken together, these various approaches combine to give you the confidence and the know how to share what you do.

Summary

Based on 15 years of helping nurses dare to share, each chapter in this example-filled guidebook, opens with real-life stories of nurses like you and closes with exercises to make each small step of the process your own. Depending on how you learn best, you can work through the exercises in this guidebook individually, with a partner, or with a group.

Conclusion

Until you take the dare to share, you won't know whether you can do it. Once you see how much fun it is to share, you'll look forward to the next dare. Once you find how your sharing changes the way others think, practice, or live their lives, you may decide to make sharing a habit you never want to break. The only other thing you need to get started is something to write with so you can participate in the activities that begin and end each chapter. Enjoy the journey!

References

1. Bunkers, S. S. (2000). The nurse scholar of the 21st century. *Nursing Science Quarterly, 13*(2), 116–123.
2. Riley, J. M., Beal, J., Levi, P., & McCauseland, M. P. (2002). Revisioning nursing scholarship. *Journal of Nursing Scholarship, 34*(4), 383–389.

Small Steps to Open to Your Creativity

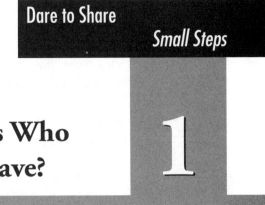

Introduction: What Do Nurses Who Dare to Share Have?

1

You gain strength, courage, and confidence by every experience in which you really stop to look fear in the face.

Eleanor Roosevelt

Let's get to the doing, you say. No frills; give me the bottom line. Just tell me how to present this idea or get that project published. Being a can-do, hands-on bunch, as nurses we want to get the techniques down first. Although know-how is essential, it's hard to overestimate the influence of inner attitude. A number of nursing texts outline the writing process; however, this guidebook is unique in exploring the personal issues that can block or boost your efforts to go public. Decide to take the dare to share and don't be surprised as fearful thoughts and bodily symptoms intrude with a persistence that can only amaze. Ignore them or pretend they're not there at your own risk. Frustration follows, momentum is stalled, and projects are abandoned and left unfinished.

What do nurses have who present and publish? A belief that they've got something special to share and a self-confidence that goes beyond the technical. Sure, they can still feel like impostors when it comes to creativity. In fact, they're on a first-name basis with their inner critics. Instead of trying to outrun them, however, these nurses expect their inner critics to show up, and they know how to handle them when they do. If you want to learn the "powerful practices" that nurses who dare to share use to propel projects forward, a shift in perspective is the first step. Then action will take on a new meaning as you make it a habit to prepare yourself for creative journeys; ask for direction from the allies you meet along the way; and play with the demons, dragons, gremlins, and goblins laying in wait.

Before you turn the page, however, a caution is in order. Even when you're open to giving the small steps introduced in this section a try, you may find yourself feeling a bit like Ralph Macchio's character in the movie *The Karate Kid*. Remember the boy whose teacher made him paint fences and wash cars when all he wanted to do was learn karate. Just as it took time for him to see that painting and polishing involve moves basic to karate, it may take awhile to appreciate how shifting your perspective on creativity and exploring your "inner landscape"[1] makes presenting and publishing possible. Be patient. Once you make the connection, you'll see that a little frustration up front is worth the pay-off in the end.

TIP
Nurses who dare to share take small steps that make for big results.

Reference

1. Palmer, P. (1990). *The courage to teach: Exploring the inner landscape of a teacher's life*. San Francisco: Jossey-Bass.

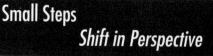
I Am a Nurse
and I Am Creative

2

*I honor the creator within me. I carry riches,
jewels, and abundance. I have a bountiful heart.
I am dowried by love, by compassion, by
companionship. I act with generosity. . . .
My creations are the creations of the creator
within me. I create with freedom and power.
I create with bliss and excitement. . . .*

Julia Cameron

If I had a penny for every time I've heard a nurse say, "I'm not creative," I could build my dream house on prime waterfront property. From expert to novice, nurses at all levels believe this. Just the other day, I was consulting with a school of nursing and the dean blurted out that she wasn't creative. A similar thing happened every semester when I told my students that their final assignment was giving creative form to a concept covered in the course. Eyes would pop and voices quiver as they squeaked, "What do you mean by creative form?" I'd always say it's your choice: Draw, sing, write a poem, make a DVD, dance. Heads would shake as each, in turn, said, "I can't do that, I'm not creative." It never failed. On the last day of class, as the originality of each project shared delighted us all, they were initiated into the secret. Nurses are creative, each in her or his own way.

Presenting and publishing are creative acts. So unless you honor the creativity within, it will be difficult to share what you do. Making this happen can be as simple as shifting your perspective. Tell yourself something new and true right now:

I am a nurse and I am creative.

To get the message to your body as well as your mind, write this new-and-true phrase five times in Jot Box 2-1.

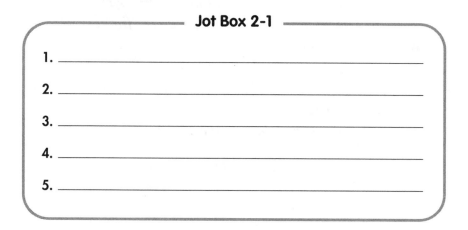

Jot Box 2-1

1. _____

2. _____

3. _____

4. _____

5. _____

Over the next few weeks, repeat this phrase silently to yourself when you're standing in line at the supermarket or when pumping gas. Or, even better, shout it out where you can't be overheard, in places like your shower or car. Yell it loud and yell it proud! If you're reading *Dare to Share* in a group or for a course, chant it aloud three times in unison, making your voices louder each time. Make it your mantra, the first and last things you say in your sessions.

Whether you're saying these simple eight words alone or together, the idea of being creative may take some getting used to. Repeat this phrase over and over and something magical might happen. Instead of feeling like an impostor, you'll begin to believe it's true—you are creative!

To help you shift your perspective, take a minute—literally—to read the question in Jot Box 2-2 and write your response to it in the space provided.

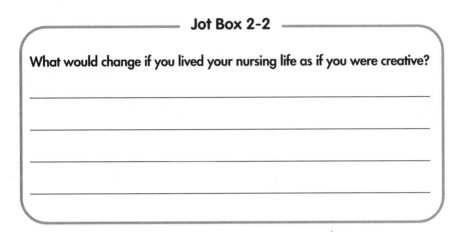

Jot Box 2-2

What would change if you lived your nursing life as if you were creative?

_____

_____

_____

_____

What would change if you lived your nursing life as a creative person? You're about to find out. The rest of the chapters in this section introduce you to four small steps that are, in essence, an action plan for nurses to get in touch with their own creativity.

TABLE 2-1 Action Plan for Each Small Step

Small Step	Action Plan
Shift in perspective	Get in a creative mood.
Self-reflect	Explore your inner landscape.
Strategies and skills	"Share-what-you-do" tools and techniques.
Support circle	Reach out to colleagues and friends.

TIP

Yes, what you say is true; you are a nurse and you are creative.

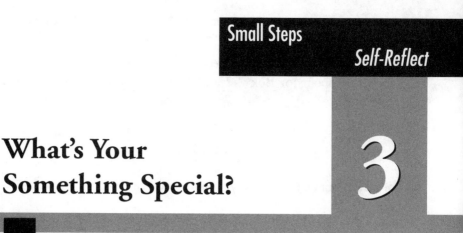

What's Your Something Special?

3

> *There is a vitality, a life force, an energy, a quickening, that is translated through you into action, and because there is only one of you in all time, this expression is unique. And if you block it, it will never exist through any other medium and will be lost.*

Martha Graham

Because there's only one of you, you bring something special to nursing. You might draw a blank, however, if I asked you to talk about your special something. I bet you'd have a story to tell if I asked you what *someone else*—a patient or a family member, a teacher, a colleague, an administrator, a student, a friend, or one of your relatives—appreciates about you as a nurse. As you read my response to the question in the following box, you might be reminded of something someone once said about you.

What's the Special Something Someone Appreciated About Me as a Nurse?

At an educator's conference in Portland, Oregon, I arrived a few minutes early for my presentation. After the handsome, dark-haired presenter finished, I began moving the chairs into a circle for my session. He approached me asking, "Are you Kathy Heinrich?" As I said yes, I glanced down at the nametag dangling from the string around my neck. Was he going to tell me that my name was upside down in the plastic holder? As he extended his hand, he said, "I'm so pleased to finally meet you. You're one of the few educators in the country who's writing about the interface between higher education and psychology."

I can still feel the warmth that surged through me when he said those words. In a single phrase—writing about the interface between education and psychology—this stranger put into words the something special that I bring to nursing. Up until then I'd been so busy merging the two that it never occurred to me that there was anything unique about it.

As I think about it now, that's what makes getting a hold of your something special a bit slippery. It is so much a part of who you are that you take it for granted; you don't see it as anything out of the ordinary. Maybe that's why it's often someone else who points out your something special.

My free-write reminded me about a pleasurable moment I hadn't thought about in a long time and gave me a new insight. Writing is an act of discovery, which is why you'll be asked to free-write your responses to questions throughout this guidebook. Take a moment to read about free-writes in Information Box 3-1.

Before you try it, let's talk about timing your free-writes. All the free-write exercises in this book are designed to take between 1 and 2 minutes. I set my egg timer for a minute when I do free-writes because a short time frame concentrates my attention. Those who find a minute too short prefer 90-second or 2-minute free-writes. Over time, you'll find the time frame that works best for you. Depending on the question being asked, you may find yourself taking a shorter or longer time to respond. As a general guideline, I'd suggest not giving yourself longer than 2 minutes for any free-write. Also, get yourself some sort of timing device so you won't have to stop in the middle of a free-write to consult your watch.

Information Box 3-1

What Is a Free-write?

Free-write exercises allocate a specified amount of time to respond to a particular question. Peter Elbow considers free-writing exercises the best way to improve your writing. Called by various names—automatic writing, babbling or jabbering exercises—free-writes allow a specified amount of time to respond to a particular question.[1] By allowing ideas to flow—no judgments, no edits—you discover what you didn't know you knew. Don't be concerned if in the beginning nothing comes to mind. Just write Xs and Os or doodle—anything to keep your pen moving. Before the time is up, ideas will begin to flow. Whether your ideas come as bullets or in complete sentences, write them down in whatever form they present themselves.

Okay, now you know all you need to write your response to the free-write question in Jot Box 3-1.

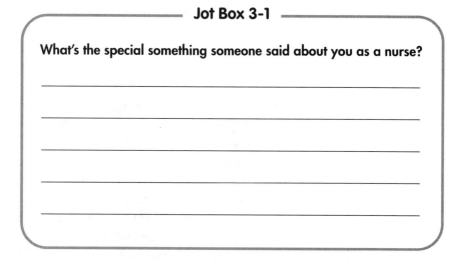

Jot Box 3-1

What's the special something someone said about you as a nurse?

_____

_____

_____

_____

_____

How was that for you? If your ideas didn't flow, be gentle with yourself; particularly if this is your first free-write. Like giving shots or drawing blood, some of the strategies and skills in this guidebook come more easily than others. With practice, you'll be amazed at how easy it is for you to complete free-writes.

> **TIP**
> For now, it's enough to hold close that memory of being seen for your something special.

Reference

1. Elbow, P. (1990). *Writing without teachers* (2nd ed.). New York: Oxford Press.

How to Recognize Your Inner Critic

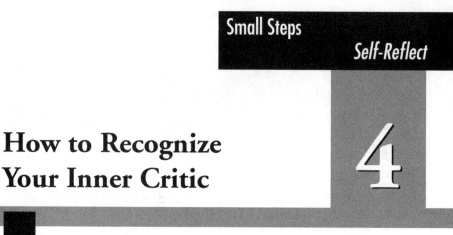

Taking a new step, uttering a new word, is what people fear the most.

Fyodor Dostoyevsky

As you were writing about your special something did you hear an inner voice whisper, "Forget about it! What's the point in getting all puffed up about something that comes as easily as breathing?" Comments like this wither your joy and jelly your innards when you even think about sharing what you do. If you think you're the only one who feels this way, think again. These inner voices, these feelings, have names. Creative writer Natalie Goldberg[1] calls this the "Inner Critic"; psychologist Peggy MacIntosh[2] calls it "the Impostor." In *Dare to Share*, the inner critic is defined as the voice your "creativity impostor" uses to keep you in line. Now that we've gotten the definitions out of the way, let's give your inner critic a name, a face, and a form.

Ever since a creative writer named Louise C. Marks made a presentation to our group about her inner critic, I knew you had to meet Griselda. So I asked Louise's permission to put words into Griselda's mouth so you can hear how she sounds. Whenever Louise faces a dare-to-share challenge, Griselda's chatter is incessant. When someone asks Louise to present, Griselda's quick to say, "You can't do that." When

Louise agrees to present, Griselda gives in, "Okay, go ahead, fall on your face, but don't say I didn't tell you so." When Louise has trouble getting started, Griselda's there to remind her, "See, I told you this was a bad idea." Under the stress of a deadline, when Louise is tempted to grab for a salty snack, Griselda coos, "Sure, eat that bag of potato chips, it'll make you feel better." When Louise feels a bit sick afterwards, Griselda cackles, "That's disgusting, now it's going to take you weeks to get the flab off your hips." If someone compliments Louise on her presentation, Griselda sniffs, "Oh, easy for them to say, they have no idea what they're talking about."

Do you have a voice like Louise's Griselda inside of you? If you kept a record of your inner critic's voice for a day, you'd hear lots of contradictory messages. You'd find out how frightened inner critics are of any change that takes them out of their comfort zone; that they're nowhere to be found when there's real danger on the horizon. Unless you really want to, there's no need to keep a record of your critic's voice for a day. You can get a read on your inner critic by completing Jot Box 4-1.

Jot Box 4-1

Whenever you think about _____ (your

next dare to share challenge), your inner critic tells you that

_____ .

When Louise asked us to give our inner critics a name, Irene O'Day, a holistic nurse in our group, named hers Judge Judy. I was stumped. It wasn't until weeks after Louise's talk when I was writing this chapter that it came to me. My inner critic has a guy's voice that's so overbearing and clunky I call him Lurch. Now it's your turn to come up with a name.

Jot Box 4-2

What is your inner critic's name?

_____

Whether or not you've got a name for your inner critic, it helps to get a visual. Griselda's got frizzy hair dyed carrot-red, pink splotches of rouge on her cheeks, and maroon lipstick running about an inch beyond and around her thin, wrinkly lips. Louise even has a doll fitting Griselda's description. I don't have a doll, but I do have a drawing of Lurch that I'd like you to see (Figure 4-1).

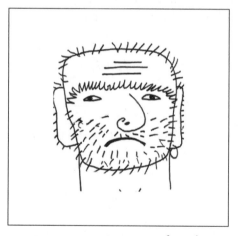

FIGURE 4-1   Drawing of Lurch

Every time I draw Lurch, no matter how scary I try to make him, he always comes out looking kind of funny and almost endearing. I used to chalk this up to my artistic limitations; now I realize that inner critics are really not as scary as they seem. Like all bullies, inner critics are afraid. No wonder being held in their grip feels like a no-win situation; they're as scared to fail as they are to succeed. Since Lurch got his name and a shape, it's easier to figure out if what I'm hearing is an inner voice with legitimate concerns or Lurch trying to intimidate me.

Now it's your turn, I've left a whole blank page for you to draw your "impostor critic" (Figure 4-2). Before you do, wait a moment and take a listen. Are you're hearing an inner voice telling you that you can't draw? Remember, this is not about being Van Gogh, it's about giving creative form to your inner critic. For once, defy your inner Griselda by having fun with this. Raid the kids' or grandkids' art supplies for crayons, colored pens, or magic markers. Gather your old magazines and make a collage mixing images and headlines. Give yourself as much time as you need for this creative assignment.

What do you notice about your drawing or collage of your inner critic? Like a virus that erupts into a red splotch on your lip when you're tired or under stress, your inner critic is most likely to show up when you're faced with a new challenge; perhaps a challenge like reading *Dare to Share*. When you notice the familiar symptoms—your throat closing, fear gripping your gut, an inner voice saying that you're crazy to think you've got something worth sharing—you'll know that your inner critic is back. That is, of course, unless your inner critic is a shape-shifter. Then, just when you figure out that a headache and the urge to escape to a tropical island are your critic's calling cards, you find that your critic has you eating everything in sight, making your stomach ache and your hips widen.

These internal voices don't go away; your inner critics are companions for life.[3] Whether consistent or a shape-shifter, over time you'll begin to recognize your critic's various voices and disguises. Although you may not be ready to join the "Hearing Voices Network,"[4] accepting the fact that you're a "recovering" impostor[5] who suffers from a chronic condition with exacerbations and remissions can be a revelation. Then, instead of dreading your critic's next appearance, you may welcome him or her as a familiar, albeit grumpy, traveling buddy.

TIP

Whenever your impostor puts in an appearance, it means that you're hot on the trail of a new adventure.

FIGURE 4-2   Drawing of Your Inner Critic

References

1. Goldberg, N. (1990). *Wild mind: Living the writer's life.* New York: Bantam Books.
2. MacIntosh, P. (1985). *Feeling like a fraud.* Working Paper No. 18. Wellesley, MA: Stone Center for Developmental Services and Studies.
3. Heinrich, K. T. (1997). Transforming impostors into heroes: metaphors for innovative nursing education. *Nurse Educator, 22*(3), 44–50.
4. Smith, D. B. (2007). *Muses, madmen, and prophets: Rethinking the history, science, and meaning of auditory hallucinations.* New York: Penguin Press.
5. Bell, L. A. (1990). The gifted woman as impostor. *Advanced Development Journal, 2,* 55–64.

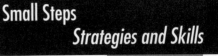

How to Take a
Creative Time-Out

5

Stalk moments of solitude.

Tillie Olson

Let me ask you a question. Would you pack your scuba diving gear for a retreat in the mountains? Of course not! Why then after a long day do you expect yourself to stumble into your workspace and design a presentation or whip out an article? And when you can't make it happen, you tell yourself that you don't have what it takes to share what you do. That's nonsense. Just as you need to pack the right stuff for a weekend getaway, you'll need to ready yourself for a creative adventure by transitioning from an active to a receptive frame of mind.

For dancers, a *still point* is a pause in the action. In *Dare to Share*, still-point strategies are simple methods for slowing the body, mind, psyche, and spirit. You're going to complete your first still-point strategy in a moment, so you'll need a private and quiet place where you won't be disturbed. If this means closing your door or moving to another room or building, do it now. When you're ready, read the instructions describing the still-point strategy in Information Box 5-1.

Information Box 5-1

A Quieting Exercise

Get into a relaxed position. Either close your eyes or focus on an object in the room. Take some deep, cleansing breaths. As you inhale, you're *breathing in* the feelings accumulated over this busy day—tension, joy, stress, satisfaction, anxiety, or happiness. As you exhale, you're *breathing out* the feelings that you need for creative work—serenity, peace, relaxation. Allow yourself to repeat this breathing in and breathing out until the bustle of the day recedes and you're in the quiet place of receptivity. Then, when you feel ready, count to three and come back to the room and open your eyes, refreshed and ready to participate. 1–2–3.

Once you've got the sequence of this breathing exercise down, give it a try.

How was that for you? When I compare how I feel now with how I felt before the quieting exercise, I know that this still-point strategy worked. When I began the exercise, I felt off-kilter. As I inhaled, I was able to put a name to what I was feeling—anxiety. By breathing in anxiety and breathing out peace, after a few inhalations and exhalations I felt at peace. Check in with how you are feeling. Are you more relaxed, about the same, more tense?

Were you surprised by the breathing instructions? You may be used to breathing out the energies that you want to release and breathing in the energies you want to attract. Tonglen breathing is just the opposite. *Tonglen* means "taking in and sending out."[1] An ancient Tibetan meditation,[2] Tonglen is a breathing practice that "activates loving-kindness and compassion"[3] by transforming "pain into compassion on the medium of your own breath."[4] If this breathing pattern quieted your mind and body, you might want to consider using it as one of your still-point strategies. If not, a new still-point strategy is shared in each section to help you find at least one that calms you.

Whatever strategy you settle on, whether it's lighting a candle, changing into comfortable clothes, or playing Baroque music, keep it simple. Let me give you an example. Diana Mixon is a nurse educator whose still-point strategy is hanging a sign on her office door whenever she's in need of a creative time-out. She played with different messages until she came up with this one: "Creativity in Progress! Would you

Interrupt God?" Being the wife of a minister, Diana's message fits her to her fingertips and keeps disturbances to a minimum.

If the very idea of solo time makes you antsy, you're not alone. Many nurses are extroverts who never spend a moment alone if they can help it. If this rings a bell, you may need some practice with taking creative time-outs, whether that means turning off the cell phone or closing your office door. There's no time like the present to start!

Create a sign with your own message. Punch a couple of holes for a string or ribbon in the upper corners so you can hang your sign on your doorknob whenever you're in need of a creative time-out. Ask family, friends, and colleagues to leave you in peace whenever they see this sign on your door. This sign, along with your request, ensures that once you make the active-receptive transition, you'll get the uninterrupted time you need for creative projects.

Even after a crazy shift, setting a still point can protect you from inner distractions as well as external interruptions Whether you have a 10-minute or 10-hour block of time to devote to a creative project, you'll notice the difference in your focus, efficiency, and productivity when you take time to shift to a receptive frame of mind.

TIP
Set a still point; take a creative time-out.

References

1. Chödrön, P. (1994). *Start where you are: A guide to compassionate living.* Boston: Shambala Press.
2. Chödrön, P. (2002). *Places that scare you.* Boston: Shambala Press.
3. Gorman, B. (2005, January/February). Gestation of compassion: Nursing education, Tonglen, and a little cello music, *Nurse Education, 30*(1), 1–3.
4. Chödrön, P., & Walker, A. (1998). *In conversation: On the meaning of suffering and the mystery of joy* [Audiotape]. Boulder, CO: Sounds True.

How Do Artist's Dates Prime Your Creativity Pump?

6

*One of the secrets of a happy life
is continuous small treats.*

Iris Murdoch

Here's a great question: When was the last time you experienced a small pleasure that made your senses come alive? I'll go first.

A Small Pleasure That Awakened My Senses

Although I like to give myself at least one small pleasure a day, I was given an amazing gift last Saturday afternoon. Weary to the bone from working on this book, I half-heartedly said yes when Chris, my significant other, asked if I wanted to go for a short walk. As we were nearing home, we saw a plastic triangle lying by the side of the road. Taking a closer look, we saw it was a sleeve holding a bouquet of fresh flowers. When we brought them home, I put them in a vase; they've turned into the most voluptuous pink and white lilies, delicate yellow and pastel pink roses, and the fattest Gerber daisies ever. With my deadline less than two weeks away, every time I see or smell these glorious petals they give me all the energy of an enthusiastic crowd cheering me on as I near the finish line.

Just writing about this bouquet brings back that sense of losing myself in the sights, smells, and soft touch of those tender petals and blooms. No wonder free-writes can be a still-point strategy.

Okay, it's your turn for a free-write (Jot Box 6-1).

Jot Box 6-1

Describe the last time you experienced a small pleasure that awakened your senses.

_____

_____

_____

_____

_____

How does your memory leave you feeling?

Many of us are so bombarded by man-made noise and external stimuli on and off the job that we shut down our senses just to make it through the day. That's why the small pleasure you just wrote about is so precious. In a world cut off from natural rhythms, it's healing for our senses whenever we create opportunities to touch, smell, see, hear, and taste in more conscious ways.[1]

Creative people stay creative by delighting their senses on a regular basis. According to Julia Cameron,[2] a mentor to all sorts of creative people, sensory pleasures keep creativity pumps primed. To indulge your small pleasures, Julia recommends taking yourself on artist's dates, which she describes as "a block of time, perhaps two hours weekly, especially set aside and committed to nurturing your creative consciousness, your inner artist . . . an excursion, a play date that you preplan and defend against all interlopers" (p. 19).[2]

To give you a better idea of an artist's date, I'll share a recent artist's date of my own. But before I do, I need to give you a bit of background.

One of the activities I loved as a child was painting. Even though I had-n't picked up a brush since I was a teenager, I got the urge to paint in my forties. I bought an easel and hundreds of dollars of art supplies that I never used; that is, until I read about a Guilford artist who'd developed a new and easy way to paint, which he calls PASTAC. Now that I've been taking art lessons with Brendan Loughlin weekly for the last three years, my artist dates often involve something related to buying art supplies or going to exhibits or art museums.

My Artist's Date

When Brendan's art was displayed in a barn-turned-studio nearby, I made that the destination for an artist's date. After seeing the paintings displayed there, I drove home by way of my favorite gelato store and lingered over a triple-chocolate gelato on a bench in the shadow of a 300-year-old tree.

Destination: Art gallery
Time frame: 3 hours
Cost: $3.50 + Gas
Value: Beyond words

I came back feeling as if I'd been away for 3 days rather than 3 hours. As you can see, an artist's date doesn't have to be time-consuming, far away, or costly.

Many nurses nix the idea of artist's dates because they don't have 2-hour blocks of time. You don't have to. That's why there are micro, mini, midi, and maxi artist's dates. Okay, Julia doesn't say this, but it's the only way I could sell the idea to busy nurses. Micro dates take 10 minutes or less, enough time to make a cup of tea and look out the window to daydream. Mini dates take 15 to 30 minutes, which is a perfect amount of time for a walk around the block or to read a favorite magazine. Midi dates are an hour, leaving time enough for a pedicure or a trip to the dollar store. Maxi dates are 2 hours or more, and my example showed you what this looks like.

How will you know what to do? If you're having trouble thinking up activities, do what I did: Follow your bliss back to childhood pas-sions. Articles and books on creativity are full of stories of adults who return to something they *neglected* to do that makes adulthood a second chance. My friend and colleague Mary Jo Barend, a newly retired, psychiatric nurse therapist, has taken up the flute and plays in a community band. Whether reviving a childhood pleasure or circling back to do something you'd wished you'd done but never got the chance, there's no need to wait until retirement to delight your senses.

As far as destinations, how do you pick where to go? Think about a place you would enjoy visiting, perhaps an art supply or hardware store. Here's a list of possible destinations gathered from nurses' artist's dates:

- Stationary store
- Art supply store
- Craft store
- Art gallery
- Book stores
- A place in nature
- Dollar store
- Hardware store
- Gift shop
- Fabric store
- Spa

Note that artist's dates don't have to be expensive. Give yourself an allowance to buy yourself a little something.

Now it's time to move your creativity into action. Make an artist's date with your inner creative self (Jot Box 6-2).

Jot Box 6-2

Your Artist's Date

Destination: _____

Micro, Mini, Midi, Maxi Time Frame: _____

Allowance: _____

Value: _____

What did you come up with? Does your artist's date include you and only you? It's common for nurses to want to multitask their artist's date—take the kids to the yarn store or meet a friend for lunch at a bookstore. Don't. Remember that an artist's date is time *for you to spend with you* to revitalize your senses.

Creative people commit to being creative. Do schedule a specific time for your artist's date and write it into your calendar, appointment book, or Palm Pilot. Be prepared for your creativity impostor to get nervous, for your inner critic to come up with reasons why you should postpone or cancel your date altogether. Guard your artist's date as if it was an appointment with a celebrity hair stylist or a reservation for a meal at a restaurant booked six months in advance.

TIP
Commit to priming your creativity pump; take yourself on artist's dates.

References

1. Olson, K. (2001, November–December). Tasting the wind, hearing the water. *Utne Reader: The Best of the Alternative Press*, 52–56.
2. Cameron, J. (1992). *The artist's way: A spiritual path to higher creativity. A course in discovering and recovering your creative self.* New York: A Jeremy P. Tarcher/Putnam Book.

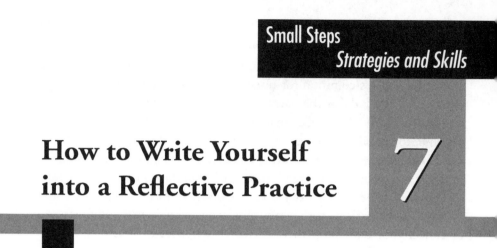

How to Write Yourself into a Reflective Practice

7

> *Writing can be used as a path to self-expression and creativity, as a path to spiritual renewal, and as a path to emotional health.*

Linda Trichter Metcalf

Nurses are action people. If health care were an athletic event, nursing would be an extreme sport. Give us a problem, and we'll deliver a plan that gets results. That's why, when asked to facilitate a journal-writing workshop with a group of emergency department nurses, I said no. I feared that they, the ultimate action figures in nursing, would laugh me out of the room when I talked about fitting time for reflection into their busy days. Only after Judy Cote, the colleague–friend who extended the invitation, assured me that they were excited about participating, did I agree to give it a try.

During the workshop, I wasn't surprised when they talked out, rather than wrote out, their answers to dialogue questions. I was amazed at how much they appreciated the opportunity to reflect on their lives and touched when they asked for a follow-up session. These men and women taught me not to judge openness to self-reflection by clinical specialty. In fact, I'm finding that the more active nurses' practices, the more they need quiet pauses and still-point moments in their days. The less they take restorative time-outs, the more at risk they are for physical, mental, emotional, and spiritual burn-outs. Although artist's dates provide pauses and moments that heal the senses, telling stories allows nurses to both delve into and get distance from the human dramas they witness and participate in every day. You may have kept your stories to yourself for so long that you need practice with telling them. Writing to yourself, exploring your inner landscape, being both storyteller and listener, is a way to begin. In addition to being a reflective practice, writing is another way to prime your creativity pump.[1] This is why I'm asking you to make your next artist's date a shopping trip to purchase a *Dare to Share* notebook.

You can find blank books and journals in many drug stores, stationary stores, bookstores, and even grocery stores. Depending on how you want to use your notebook, you can buy a pocket-sized one that you can keep with you or a regular sized one to keep at home. I keep my notebook in my pocketbook. The cover is a bouncy design of colored circles; it has a purple elastic ribbon that holds my place and thick paper that makes the pages fun to write on. This book features a number of creative assignments that require you to have a *Dare to Share* notebook, so get one you enjoy writing in because you're going to be using it a lot.

When you begin by writing your stories to yourself, it's a shorter distance to sharing them with others. What are presentations and publications but storytelling? So start private. Use your notebook for reflective free-writes, meditations on your practice, personal insights, working though issues and conflicts with others or for recording drawings, sayings, and poems. In the process, you may find yourself morphing from action figure to reflective practitioner to public speaker and author.

TIP

To share what you do, you must reflect on what you do.

References

1. Cameron, J. (1992). *The artist's way: A spiritual path to higher creativity. A course in discovering and recovering your creative self.* New York: A Jeremy P. Tarcher/Putnam Book.

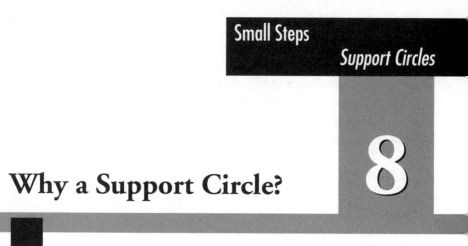

Why a Support Circle?

8

*Call it a clan, call it a network, call it a tribe,
call it a family. Whatever you call it, whoever
you are, you need one.*

Jane Howard

The idea of reaching out to allies, helpers, and rooters may be as alien to you as putting a sign on your door, taking yourself on an artist's date, or writing about your inner landscape. Even though we're there for everyone else, nurses tend to go it alone rather than ask for help. If you want to dare to share, this is going to have to change. Although up until now we've been talking about creativity as a solo act, no human creation has ever been accomplished alone. Think about writers like Hemingway and artists like Picasso. Their lives intertwined alone time creating in their studios and hanging out with creative others in cafes, restaurants, and bars. Enriched and fortified by these interchanges, they'd return to their studios to build upon or break away from what others were thinking and doing, their relationships inspiring and being inspired by their creativity.

To give you a sense of what support circles feel like, you'll be making this dare-to-share journey with three nurse companions. Although they may sound like you or your colleagues, their stories are composites of the nurses I've known and learned from over the last 30 years. Meet

Keri, Betty, and Justin and learn about what they hope to get from *Dare to Share*.

Keri, a Native American who just graduated from a second degree program where she got a baccalaureate and master's degree in three years introduces herself by saying:

> My Indian name means "bird in flight." Maybe that's why I couldn't wait to get away from the "res." As soon as I could, I got myself into Berkeley where I majored in anthropology. After finishing, I realized that I wanted to help people in a more hands-on way than my degree allowed for, so I decided to become a nurse. This year, on my 29th birthday, I opened my practice as a nurse practitioner on the same reservation I flew away from a little more than 10 years ago. My master's thesis explored the challenges Native Americans face in providing health care to their own people. I'm reading *Dare to Share* to find out how to turn my 100-page thesis into an article for nurse practitioners.

Betty's colleague, Colleen, introduces her and explains how Betty ended up reading this book:

> Betty graduated from her community hospital's diploma program in 1965. In between raising three children, she's worked at "her" hospital ever since. The flowers from her garden brighten our unit in the summer; her tomatoes and green squash make great sauces and breads for Christmas presents that come with best wishes to stay warm during our Midwestern winters. She's always knitting a sweater for a niece or sewing a quilt for someone who's retiring. A great listener, I've watched Betty spend hours helping co-workers find ideas for presentations that make their eyes glitter. Whenever Betty edits my manuscripts, she's always sensitive to my feelings. She asks insightful questions and makes suggestions for changes. Yet Betty has never presented or published her own work. When I've asked why not, she always says, "What with helping everybody else, I don't really have the time." I gave Betty a copy of *Dare to Share* in hopes that she'll do for herself what she's been doing for the rest of us.

Justin is 35 years old, husband and father of a 5-year-old son, and a baccalaureate nursing student, who says:

> I was naïve thinking that my gender wouldn't affect how I was treated as a nurse. During my associate degree program, I became aware of the challenges of being a man in a profession traditionally made up of women. When I entered my baccalaureate program, I got the men together to discuss challenges of being a man in a women's profession and suggested that we meet regularly. They voted me president and we call ourselves, "Men in Nursing." In our group, we help one another with everything from tutoring to strategizing how to deal with tricky interpersonal interactions with everyone from patients to administrators.
>
> I picked up *Dare to Share* because speaking at conferences and writing articles is the best way to get our group recognized as a chapter by the national organization. Going public will also help me advocate for attracting men into nursing and supporting them during and following their educational experiences.

At the beginning of each section you'll be able to measure your own dreams and challenges against theirs. In the conclusion to each section you'll realize how much you've learned by reading about what they've learned about daring to share.

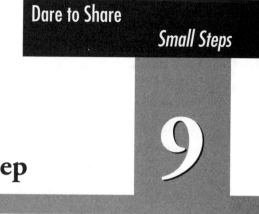

Conclusion: Commit to a Creative Next Step

Will you be a hero in your daily work?

Florence Nightingale

Sharing what you do is a creative act. In this section, you've learned that you're creative in your own special way. You've even answered the question: "What would change if you lived your nursing life as if you were creative?" For your nursing companions, free-writing their answer to this question really did shift their perspective.

Keri wrote:

> If I lived my nursing life as if I were creative, I'd be keeping a journal of my daily experiences as a nurse practitioner new to practice and new to being among my people as a professional helper rather than as a dependent child.

Keri's scheduled an artist's date this coming week to buy herself a *Dare to Share* notebook.

Betty's free-write read:

> To live my life as a creative nurse, I'm going to have to stand up to Desiree, my inner critic. She looks beautiful and sounds lovely whenever I'm taking care of others. Things get ugly whenever I take time to do something for myself.

Betty does want to share what she does at least once before she retires. So she's taking her *Dare to Share* notebook to a nearby café for a latte and a brainstorming session.

Justin wrote:

> To live out my creativity as a nurse will include presenting and publishing articles about increasing the number as well as the respect for men in nursing.

Justin is committing himself to developing an idea for a presentation on this topic in the next section.

To refresh your memory, the 15 powerful practices discussed in Section 1 are summarized in Information Box 9-1.

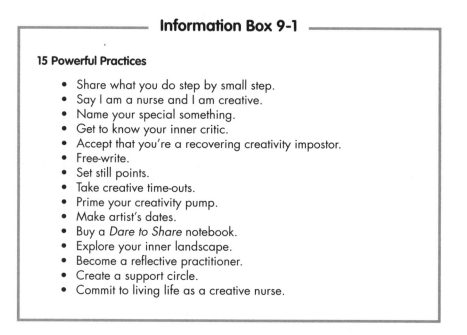

Information Box 9-1

15 Powerful Practices

- Share what you do step by small step.
- Say I am a nurse and I am creative.
- Name your special something.
- Get to know your inner critic.
- Accept that you're a recovering creativity impostor.
- Free-write.
- Set still points.
- Take creative time-outs.
- Prime your creativity pump.
- Make artist's dates.
- Buy a *Dare to Share* notebook.
- Explore your inner landscape.
- Become a reflective practitioner.
- Create a support circle.
- Commit to living life as a creative nurse.

Now that you've read your nurse companions' commitments and scanned the 15 Powerful Practices, it's your turn to commit to a creative next step (use Jot Box 9-1).

Jot Box 9-1

I commit to the next creative step of

_____

_____

_____

_____

_____

Congratulations! Now that you've committed yourself to a creative next step, you're ready to learn more about presenting what you do.

TIP
Creative people commit to doing creative things.

Small Steps to Present What You Do

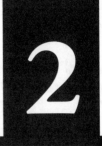

Introduction: How Are Presentations Defined?

10

In this high place
It is as simple as this
Leave everything you know behind.

David Whyte

Because nurses are always presenting information, both informally and formally, presentations are defined broadly. A presentation may be a guest lecture in someone else's course; a storytelling session you're hosting for your hospital's Nurse's Day celebration; a workshop session for a professional group; or a formal poster presentation at a national conference. No matter what, when, and where you're presenting, are you looking forward to it or do you dread the very idea? Whether you're excited or fretful about presenting, not knowing where to go next stops many nurses from presenting what they do.

With this section serving as your presenter-mentor, you'll develop your own presentation small step by small step, from stalking eye-glittering ideas to brainstorming irresistible slants to assessing audience response. After shifting to "Beginner's Mind," you'll learn to capitalize on your presenting style; tailor your topic to your audience by using the Presentation Worksheet; engage participants through interactive learning celebrations; reach out to colleague–friends as co-presenters and peer mentors; design presentation packets; create PowerPoint slide presentations; and refine presentations based on participants' feedback. Two real-life examples of presentations that couldn't be more different—one a professional development session and the other a poster presentation—show you how.

Before discussing the concept of beginner's mind, let's check in with your three nurse companions. Read each one's response to the free-write question, "What would you like to take away from this section on presenting?"

Keri wrote:

> I'm keeping a daily log of reflections on my practitioner practice in my *Dare to Share* notebook. I'm wondering if I can use my entries as the "database" for a poster presentation on the developmental stages that I, as a Native American nurse practitioner, experienced in my first year of practice on the reservation where I grew up.

Betty's free-write reads:

> After my brainstorming session at my favorite café, which was a lovely artist's date I might add, no matter what my inner critic Desiree says, I've decided to submit a proposal to present a session on tips for nurse colleagues mentoring each other to present and publish at our hospital's next Nurse's Day celebration.

Justin wrote:

> I'd like to come away from this section with a presentation proposal, either for a poster or paper, related to our "Men in Nursing" group.

All three of your nurse companions are toying with the idea of turning their everyday experiences into presentations. To find out where you are with presenting, give yourself a minute to complete the free-write question in Jot Box 10-1.

Jot Box 10-1

What would you like to take away from this section on presenting?

_____

_____

_____

_____

Whether presenting is your life's goal or something you're doing for a grade or to keep your job, after reading this section you'll know how to make a topic so intriguing that your audience participants won't want to leave. Novice or expert, there are lessons to be learned in this section. The first is to keep your beginner's mind.

TIP
Consider presenting as a way to share what you do.

I Bring Beginner's Mind to My Life as a Nurse

11

In the beginner's mind there are many possibilities, in the expert's mind there are few.

Shunryu Suzuki

After hearing thousands of dreams over the years, Carl Jung listened to each one as if it were the first dream he'd ever heard. Buddhists call this beginner's mind.[1] To learn more about beginner's mind, give yourself a couple of minutes to read and reread the following passage. Instead of speed-reading, take the time to savor each word. Ask yourself questions. Read the ideas and phrases right side up, sideways, and upside down:

> The mind of the beginner is empty, free of the habits of the expert, ready to accept, to doubt, and open to all the possibilities . . . In the beginner's mind there is no thought, "I have attained something." All self-centered thoughts limit our vast mind. When we have no thought of achievement, no thought of self, we are true beginners. Then we can really learn something. The beginner's mind is the mind of compassion. When our mind is compassionate, it is boundless . . . Then we are always true to ourselves, in sympathy with all beings . . . So

the most difficult thing is always to keep your beginner's mind (pp.14, 21, 22).[1]

What did you learn from meditating on this passage? From your first nursing course, you've worked hard to learn all there is to know about nursing. We all know, and Patricia Benner's[2] research proved it, that nurses progress from novice to experts over the course of their professional lives. The paradox is that the more expert you are, the more difficult it is to keep a beginner's mind. Consider your answer to the question in Jot Box 11-1 as you read my response.

What would change if I lived my nursing life with beginner's mind?

Living with beginner's mind would have me asking questions, never assuming that I know anything with the smugness of the expert. Curious and in the moment, my wide-eyed enthusiasm and a spontaneity would break through preconceived molds of mind as fresh as a flower bursting forth from the seam of a crack in a stone wall..

Now it's your turn to shift your perspective by free-writing your response to the same question (Jot Box 11-1).

Jot Box 11-1

What would change if you lived your nursing life with beginner's mind?

_____

_____

_____

_____

_____

If you wrote about keeping your perspective fresh, your mind open to new possibilities, and your imagination playful, you're in beginner's mind territory.

Commit to reading this section with beginner's mind and you'll get lots of practice as you explore your inner landscape as a presenter and translate your eye-glittering idea into a presentation that makes your participants' eyes glitter.

TIP
Whether this is the first or the 100th time that you've presented what you do, keep a beginner's mind.

References

1. Suzuki, S. (1982). *Zen mind, beginner's mind: Informal talks on Zen meditation and practice*. New York: John Weatherhill.
2. Benner, P. (1983). *From novice to expert*. Menlo Park, CA: Addison-Wesley.

What's Your Preference as a Learner?

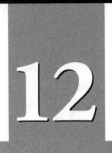

*The most profound relationship
we'll ever have is with ourselves.*

Shirley Maclaine

Laura, an advanced practice nurse, approached me after a presentation I gave about using public speaking as an advertising tool. She wanted to use presentations to advertise her practice in a holistic nurses' collective but she put herself through hell every time she tried. For weeks, she'd read everything she could find on a topic. A few days before the presentation, she was so nerved up that she'd given herself a migraine. By the day of, she couldn't get from one side of her office to the other because the floor was a chaos of books and articles. Up until the moment she took the podium, Laura was still reshuffling her note cards. Could I help her? I wasn't sure, but I said I'd give it a try.

When we met at the café that overlooks our town green, I asked Laura to tell me about a presenter she admires. She told me about Bob, a man in her graduating class, who holds audiences rapt with his lectures. She herself feels most comfortable asking questions that engage audiences in discussing ideas among themselves. "But that isn't really presenting, is it?" Laura asked with head bowed, eyes downcast. That's when I knew I could help her. Worse than making herself sick trying to imitate Bob, Laura didn't know that her presentation style has a name.

43

As you read about the stories I told Laura about three presenters' styles, pick the one that most appeals to you *as a learner*.

Samantha is a vivacious, blue-eyed redhead who engages audiences, the bigger the better, with funny stories, rapid-fire comebacks, and thorough explanations of theoretical constructs. As she sees it, her role as the presenter is to stay in control of the learning that takes place. Samantha prepares by outlining her presentations point-by-point. It's important to her that she covers all the items on her outline to ensure that her audience learns the content necessary for them to understand her work.

Tom is a quiet man with dark hair and eyes the color of the cappuccinos he drinks. He enjoys engaging small groups of participants in dialogue. Viewing his role as that of a facilitator, Tom comes prepared with a few open-ended questions. Rather than controlling the information content and flow, he prefers to allow learning to emerge from the points and counterpoints discussed. He makes the learning relevant by connecting participants' questions with conceptual ideas drawn from his working knowledge gleaned from reading widely.

Beth is a blond-haired woman with a dancer's body who prides herself on being able to tune into her audience-participants' learning needs. She shifts easily from lecture to dialogue. To prepare, Beth outlines key points and formulates thought-provoking questions. During the learning experience, she goes with the flow, balancing out controlling what's learned and allowing learning to happen.

After hearing about all three presenters, Laura wrote her answer to the question in Jot Box 12-1.

Jot Box 12-1

Whose presenting style do you prefer as a learner and why?

I very much enjoy an entertaining lecturer like Samantha. No matter how great a lecturer, I inevitably find myself getting restless because I want to know what others in the audience think. When there's no time for dialogue or audience involvement, I leave presentations feeling let down. So it's not Samantha's lecture that most appeals to me as a learner. I prefer interactive learning experiences facilitated by a Beth who moves easily between sharing information like Samantha and facilitating like Tom.

Before Laura shared what she wrote, I would have guessed that her favorite style was Samantha's. We were both surprised when she chose Beth's style that alternates between lecturing and facilitating dialogues.

Now it's your turn to put pen to paper. Is it Samantha, Tom, or Beth's style that most appeals to you as a learner (Jot Box 12-2)?

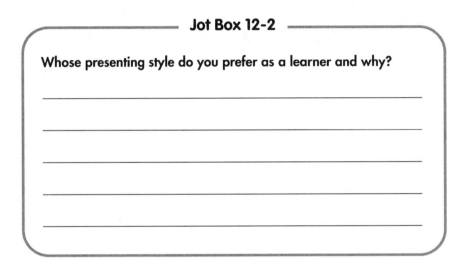

Jot Box 12-2

Whose presenting style do you prefer as a learner and why?

When it comes to presenting styles, adult educators talk about Sages-on-the-Stage and Guides-on-the-Side. Matching presenting styles to faces, Samantha is a Sage and Tom is a Guide. I've added a third style—the Best-of-Both (B.O.B.)—to describe Beth's style, which combines both Sage and Guide strategies. Because Laura's preference is Beth's, the style she prefers as a learner is a Best-of-Both. Check the presenting style that best describes your preference in Jot Box 12-3.

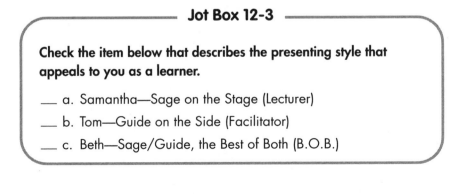

Jot Box 12-3

Check the item below that describes the presenting style that appeals to you as a learner.

___ a. Samantha—Sage on the Stage (Lecturer)

___ b. Tom—Guide on the Side (Facilitator)

___ c. Beth—Sage/Guide, the Best of Both (B.O.B.)

Once Laura figured out the style she prefers in presenters, she wanted to learn more about her own presenting style. After reading the next two chapters, you'll know more about your strengths and challenges as a presenter.

TIP
Your preference as a learner offers a glimpse into your presenting style.

What's Your Something Special as a Presenter?

13

The question we most commonly ask is the "what" question—what subjects shall we teach? . . . But seldom if ever do we ask the "who" question— who is the self that teaches?

Parker Palmer

When's the last time you shared information about your area of expertise with someone, whether it was a neighbor or a professional colleague? If it wasn't today, it was yesterday. While these may not be formal prsentations, they do involve your sharing what you know with others. As staff nurses or advanced practice nurses, you meet with patients and their families, round with physicians, and give report at change of shift. As educators and administrators, you make informal and formal presentations to small and large groups on a daily basis. As nurse entrepreneurs, you present every time you speak about your business. Your approach, the one that you've developed over time, is your "something special" as a presenter.

Finding the words to describe this something special is far from a vanity exercise; it helps you name your presenting style. Knowing this name may not make putting your something special as a presenter into words any easier. That's why it's often someone else—a mentor, a colleague, or an audience participant—who puts words around your gifts as a presenter. For me, it was a colleague's observation that captured my essence as a presenter.

What's my something special as a presenter?

My something special as a presenter is my ability to reach out and create an intimate connection with audiences.

Before you answer this "something special" question, use the list of presenter's gifts in Information Box 13-1 as a cheat sheet.

Information Box 13-1

List of Presenter's Gifts

Well-organized
Energetic
Passionate
Exuberant
Clear communicator
Accessible
Warm
Compassionate
Punctual
Creative
Engaging storyteller
Funny
Flexible
Knowledgeable
Technically proficient
Considerate
Thought-provoking
Distinctive
Interactive

If you're still not sure how to describe your special something, look at evaluations from previous presentations to see what words participants use to describe your style. Or ask colleagues who have seen you present. If you're shy about asking face-to-face, e-mail them, asking what they most appreciate about you as a presenter. It's as fun as it is affirming to read what they write back.

The last option doesn't require asking anyone anything. You have an internal observer who is balanced and objective. Enlist your internal observer to watch as you share information with others over the next few days. At the end of that time, devote an entry in your *Dare to Share* notebook asking how your internal observer would describe your special something as a presenter. Writing to inner figures, from internal observers to characters in dreams, is called "active imagination."[1] After you get over feeling funny about writing to people that others can't see, you'll be amazed at what you can learn.

However you get the information, whenever you're ready, answer the question in Jot Box 13-1 *in pencil.*

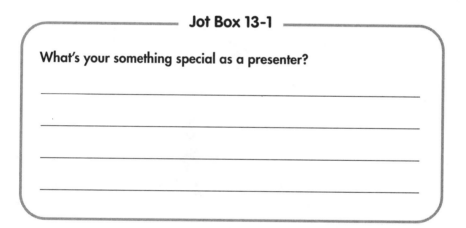

Jot Box 13-1

What's your something special as a presenter?

Take a moment to reread what you just wrote. You'll know you've got it right when rereading your free-write leaves you sighing with the satisfaction of recognition. If your response isn't yet in the "essence zone," that's fine. It can take years to find an answer that's spot-on, which is why you wrote your answer in pencil. Even when you find the perfect description, it may change. In a couple of months or a year from now, you'll replace what you wrote with something entirely different. So enjoy the search and expect insights to come from unexpected sources.

> **TIP**
> Keep your written description of your something special as a presenter displayed in a place where you can see it.

References

1. Hannah, B. (1981). *Active imagination: Encounters with the soul: As developed by C. G. Jung.* Fort Collins, CO: Sigo Press.

What's Your Presenting Style?

Cherish forever what makes you unique,
'cuz you're really a yawn if it goes!

Bette Midler

Keep in mind what you've learned about your special something as you complete the quiz in Jot Box 14-1.

Jot Box 14-1

Your Presenting Style Checklist

___1. I shine when I'm center-stage performing in the spotlight.

___2. I prefer to shine the spotlight on others by asking them questions.

___3. I enjoy the opportunity to share my knowledge with others.

___4. I want to share information related to participants' interests.

___5. I am most comfortable with the lecture style of presenting.

___6. I feel most comfortable with a facilitation style that fosters dialogue.

If you checked items 1, 3, and 5, then you're a "Sage on the Stage." You enjoy entertaining your audience by lecturing from a preplanned outline of informational points. If you checked items 2, 4, and 6, then you're a "Guide on the Side." You engage participants in a dialogue that surfaces relevant concepts and theoretical points. If you checked items 1 through 6, then you're a "Best of Both." Depending on your audience's learning needs, you switch from lecture to dialogue and back again. Check off your presenting-style preference in Jot Box 14-2.

Jot Box 14-2

Your presenting-style preference is:

___ a. Sage on the Stage (lecturer)

___ b. Guide on the Side (facilitator)

___ c. Best of Both (lecturer and facilitator)

Famous artists develop styles so uniquely their own that their artwork is immediately recognizable as a Picasso, a Renoir, or a Van Gogh. Now that you know what your special something is, you can develop a presenting style that becomes your signature. To round out your appreciation of your style, in the next chapter you'll explore your challenges as a presenter.

TIP

Appreciate the presenting style that's distinctly yours.

What's Your Greatest Challenge as a Presenter?

15

And the trouble is, if you don't risk anything,
you risk even more.

Erica Jong

What's your greatest challenge as a presenter? If you're not sure, it's time to play the opposites game. Your greatest challenge is the flip side of your special something. To show you what I mean, let's review Laura's responses to the items in Jot Box 15-1.

Jot Box 15-1

What's your special something as a presenter?
Engaging audiences in a dialogue.
What's your presenting style?
Guide-on-the-Side.
What's your greatest challenge as a presenter?
Overwhelming participants with too many theories.

Laura's concern about overwhelming participants is the flip side of her special something of engaging audiences. How does this relate to her being a Guide? Whereas Sages can overlook audiences by overemphasizing the importance of theoretical content, Guides can overlook theoretical content by overemphasizing their relationship with participants. When this occurs, Guides may either overdo or neglect theory. Only B.O.B.s value content and participants in equal measure. These three types of presenters differ in their *audience awareness*; that is, the extent to which they take attendees into account in the design, delivery, and assessment of their presentations (see Table 15-1).

TABLE 15-1 Comparison of Three Presenters' Styles

	Value	Special Something	Challenge
Sage	Theory	Communicate information	Audience awareness
Guide	Relationship	Engage in dialogue	Stating own views
B.O.B.	Theory/relationship	Alternate theory/dialogue	Use styles selectively

Low on audience awareness, Sages focus on what *they* think is important for audiences to know. They fear audiences asking questions that divert them from covering the content they've so carefully outlined. Because they like being seen as experts, they're also concerned that audiences will ask questions that they won't know how to answer. Audience aware, Guides' greatest challenge is stating an idea or an opinion before they know where their participants stand. B.O.B.s' are challenged to become more selective in their use of lecture and dialogue.

Now that you understand more about the challenges for each style, take a minute to identify your special something, style, and challenge as a presenter in Jot Box 15-1.

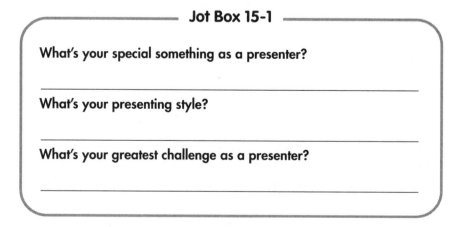

Jot Box 15-1

What's your special something as a presenter?

_____

What's your presenting style?

_____

What's your greatest challenge as a presenter?

_____

When Laura first learned about Sages and Guides, she laughingly diagnosed herself as a Guide with Sage-envy. You envy what you want to become. Said another way, your greatest challenge points the direction for your growth as a presenter. If you're a Sage, you'll never be a Guide, or vice-versa. What you can do is develop the qualities that you admire/envy in presenters whose style is different than yours. Sages will want to raise their audience awareness; Guides will want to develop a greater comfort with being experts and stating their own ideas or opinions; B.O.B.s will want to become more selective in their use of Sage and Guide styles.

Laura's free-write shows you how to reframe your presenter's challenge by translating it into a future direction (Jot Box 15-2).

Jot Box 15-2

As a _Guide,_ my future direction as a presenter _is to develop my Sage-like ability to boil theory down to a few key points._

Now it's your turn to fill in the blank:

Jot Box 15-3

As a _____ (your presenting style), your

future direction as a presenter is to develop your ability to

_____.

Whatever their particular challenge, many nurses want to develop a style that appeals to all audiences by combining Sage and Guide qualities. Before you're introduced to a learning model that makes this possible, the next chapter addresses the shyness challenge.

TIP

Your greatest challenge points the direction to your future development as a presenter.

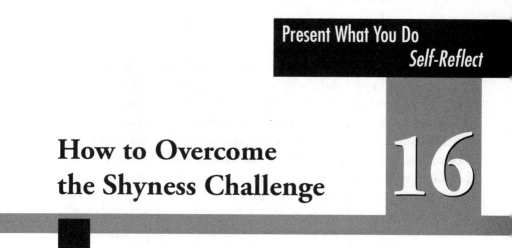

How to Overcome the Shyness Challenge

16

When I dare to be powerful, to use my strength in the service of my vision, then it becomes less and less important whether I am afraid.

Audre Lorde

If you're a shy person, should you forget about presenting? Not a chance. Shy people present all the time, as you can see from this snippet from an article about television personality Meredith Vieira:

> When asked for tales of her own, she answers simply and then deflects with a question. Her explanation is one that so many smooth, self-possessed people give and that the rest of us rarely believe: She is shy. Yes, she talked about her sex life and her children, and pretty much anything on *The View,* but that she insists, was "in character," and when the camera is off, she clearly would rather listen (p. 24).[1]

Being "in character" transforms Meredith from a quiet listener into someone who shares personal details with thousands of viewers.

What happens when Meredith steps in front of the camera? Who knows. What I do know is that shy people can present because I'm one of them. When a conference convener called to ask if I could make a kick-off session interactive for a conference audience of 1,000 nurse educators, the pause was so long that she must have thought we'd lost our connection. In a sense we had. I was distracted by an internal tug-of-war caught between Lurch screeching, "Are you crazy? You do best with audiences of 10. Don't say yes or you'll just make yourself a wreck beforehand. Then, when you bomb out, it'll be in front of an audience of 1,000 of your colleagues." And a soft and confident voice that countered, "Don't listen to him, he's just afraid. He wants to protect you but you don't need that kind of protection anymore. You're ready. You can do this!" I have no idea where this voice came from, but it must have been convincing, because the next thing I heard myself saying was, "Yes. How kind of you to think of me. Of course, I can make this session experiential." That quiet inner voice was right. I was ready *and* this was one of most satisfying, albeit scariest, things I've ever done.

To morph from shy person to presenter, I imagine myself putting on a mask like an actor in one of those Greek plays. Called a *persona*,[2] donning this mask turns me into a public speaker. Persona off, in my everyday life I'm awkward with people I don't know, I can't remember the punch lines of jokes, and my stories get bogged down with too many details. Persona on, I access a part of me that's alert, confident, funny, connected, and quick on my feet. No longer shy, I become my best and extroverted, social self. When I present, I prune stories until they contain only the details that underscore the point I'm trying to make. So my signature storytelling that may seem effortless to audiences is actually a combination of persona and practice.

Before a presentation, donning my presenter's persona is as crucial as putting on my lucky outfit—the one I wear on those days when I can do no wrong. What qualities does my presenter's persona allow me to access?

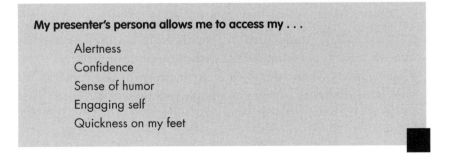

My presenter's persona allows me to access my . . .

Alertness

Confidence

Sense of humor

Engaging self

Quickness on my feet

Call it what you will—faking it until you make it, acting more confident than you feel—if you're shy, your persona can make presenting possible and even enjoyable. If you consider yourself to be shy in front of audiences, answer the question in Jot Box 16-1.

Jot Box 16-1

What qualities does your presenter's persona help you to access?

_____

_____

_____

Your presenter's persona can help bridge the gap between your private and public self. Is this mask a shy person's confidence trick? When I asked Karen Owen, an outgoing, school nurse colleague, if she needs a persona to present, she said no. Extroverts show their best side to the world so their persona is almost always in place. What Karen did say is that extroverts cannot depend on charm to carry off their presentations. So, whether or not you need a persona to present, you do need to prepare and practice.

A presenter's persona can bridge the gap between your private and your public self. Now that you know that being shy doesn't have to hold you back, you're ready to learn how to present what you do.

TIP

Don't let shyness get in your way, put on your persona and present what you do.

References

1. Belkin, L. (2006, August 13). Her morning shift. *The New York Times Magazine*. Section 6, p. 24.
2. Jung, C. G. (1959). The archetypes and the collective unconscious. *The collected works of C.G. Jung* (Vol. 9). New York: Pantheon Books.

How to Get Physical with Your Still-Point Strategy

*I only went out for a walk and finally
concluded to stay out 'til sundown,
for going out, was really going in.*

John Muir

When Karen Owen, the extroverted nurse from Chapter 16, agreed to be my peer mentor, we set a time to walk *and* talk about designing my presentation. Walking, whether you're talking or not, is a great way to unravel dilemmas, work out ideas, and hatch plans. Even if you're not collaborating with a colleague–friend, try going physical with your still-point strategy! Do some stretching before sitting down at the computer. Straighten up your workspace. Climb up and down your stairs a few times; dance around the kitchen to get into a creative mood.

When we spoke about still-point strategies in Section 1, you may not have thought about these pauses in physical terms. Once you try it out, you may find that your favored still-point strategy is some form of exercise, whether it's a tennis game or a stroll along the beach. As described in the following box, physical exercise was essential to my establishing a still point while writing *Dare to Share*.

What's My Favorite Physical Way to Create a Still Point?

Since I've been spending four to eight hours a day writing, I've found that I need at least one to two hours of dance or exercise a day as a balance to reading, composing, or revising. My favorite exercises for creating still point includes walking, as well as Pilates, yoga, and weight lifting classes. After working out, I find it easier to settle down to that day's writing tasks with much less muss and fuss, procrastination, and agitation.

You may be thinking that you're not a physical person; that exercise is one of those "me" activities lost in the chaos of busy days. Even when you are open to making your still point physical, you may not be sure which activity to choose. Not to worry. Before you answer the same question I just answered, scan the activities listed in Information Box 17-1.

Information Box 17-1

Physical Activities

    Outdoor Activities
    Walking
    Running
    Hiking
    Snowshoeing
    Skiing
    Biking
    Golfing
    Surfing

    Indoor Activities
    Cleaning
    Shopping
    Stretching
    Yoga
    Pilates
    Dancing
    Step class
    Spinning
    Weight lifting

As the muscles in your limbs warm up and your endorphins flow, you may find your mind unraveling tangles of problems and flooding with creative ideas. No wonder! Physical exercise calms bodies and concentrates minds to set imaginations free. Growing evidence suggests that physical activity makes us smarter by growing new nerve cells, causing older cells to form webs that make the brain run more efficiently, and even staving off the beginnings of Alzheimer's disease, ADHD, and other cognitive disorders.[1] So there's lots of good reasons to use a physical still-point strategy to shift to a reflective frame of mind by being active. Now that you've given it a bit of thought, write your response in Jot Box 17-1.

Jot Box 17-1

What's your favorite physical way to create a still point?

_____

_____

_____

Some still-point strategies work better than others, so give yourself time to experiment. You may, for example, find that hiking works and kickboxing doesn't, or that neither works and yoga is the way for you to go physical. Then, no matter what you decide about physical still points, you will have considered a range of possibilities. If you do find one or two physical still-point strategies that work for you, that's great! When collaborating with a peer mentor or co-presenter, you may want to ask them to share some physical activity as a playful prelude to embarking on a shared creative project.

TIP

Be sure to include physical activity in your repertoire of standard still-point strategies.

Reference

1. Carmichael, M. (2007, March 26). Stronger, faster, smarter. Health for Life. *Newsweek,* 38–46.

How to Divide Your Presentation Project into Steps

18

Sow an act, and reap a habit. Sow a habit, and you reap a character. Sow a character and you reap a destiny.

Charles Reade

What if you didn't have a standard set of steps for conducting a physical examination? As with any procedure, in the case of designing presentations it's best to set out a sequence of steps to follow before initiating the planning process. Information box 18-1 details the sequence of steps that I follow when developing my presentations.

Each of the chapters in this Strategies and Skills section is devoted to a single small step. After you select an eye-glittering idea, you'll learn to use what's called the Presentation Worksheet to attend to the elements essential to an effective presentation. Using the example of one of my recent presentations to a group of school nurses, you'll learn to translate this procedural punch list into a time line with specific dates and deadlines to keep your project on track.

Information Box 18-1

---

13 Small Steps for Presentations

1. Settle on an eye-glittering idea.
2. Complete a Presentation Worksheet to identify the following:
   - Idea/topic/focus
   - Purpose
   - Audience
   - Venue
   - Desired audience response
3. Conduct a literature search.
4. Line up a peer mentor.
5. Return to Presentation Worksheet to identify the following:
   - Slant.
   - One-sentence description.
6. Kolb your presentation.
7. Create a presentation packet.
8. Design a PowerPoint slide display.
9. Meet with your peer mentor for a preconference session.
10. Revise presentation, packet, and PowerPoint slides.
11. Present.
12. Assess your presentation:
   - Collate audience evaluations.
   - Identify what worked and what didn't work.
13. Meet with your peer mentor for a post-conference session.

When you reach the end of this section, you will know how to design a presentation using this sequence of steps.

TIP

Stay focused, on time, and on track by completing a Presentation Time Line Worksheet.

How to Find the Ideas in Your Challenges

19

*[Presentations]. . . start with a vision
of the possible or a problematic.*

Lee Shulman

Have you ever wondered where nurse presenters find such great ideas? When I asked a class of school nurses to identify a challenge in their practice, Ann's free-write read:

> I work with middle-school children. I can tell when fifth graders are having trouble keeping up with the changes in their bodies because their hygiene suffers. It's embarrassing for us both when a kid comes into my office and I notice an odor that shouldn't be there or they get referred by a teacher with a request that I speak to them about cleaning up their act. I want to develop a humorous, interactive presentation on good hygiene that can be given to all the fifth grade classes and repeated yearly with new classes.

As you can see, Ann's free-write identified a single idea. The problem she started out with—fifth graders' poor hygiene practices secondary to physical changes—became a vision of the possible—a fun and interactive presentation.

How can you find a single idea that's intriguing enough to commit to turning it into a presentation? Like Ann, start with what you know and scan your everyday experiences for ideas. When you *think presentations*, ideas will pop up in the midst of conversations, while reading or reflecting on your practice. When you're on the lookout, you'll begin to see the ideas all around you.

Whether it's a problem or a vision of the possible, find an idea that involves something or someone that you care about. Start with the challenges you're facing in your work life by completing the free-write in Jot Box 19-1.

Jot Box 19-1

What challenge(s) are you facing in your practice that makes your eyes glitter or that keeps you awake at night?

_____

_____

_____

_____

_____

_____

So what happened? Is the Jot Box empty? Does it contain a single challenge? Or does it contain an overflow of challenges? Don't worry if you had trouble identifying a challenge. Just as you may have needed more time to observe your style, you may need a week or so to hunt and gather, track and stalk, eye-glittering challenges. If you identified a single challenge with ease, that's great. If your Jot Box is stuffed with 10 different challenges, you'll learn how to pare down your list to a single challenge in the next chapter.

No matter how many or few, your challenges are a rich source of presentable ideas. These ideas can be as elusive as dream images; so unless you find a way to record them, you'll forget them. That's why journalists keep a pad and pen in a back pocket; whenever inspiration strikes, they're ready. This is where your *Dare to Share* notebook can come in handy. Until now, you may have been using it as a reflection journal. Notebooks can also be used to keep a running list of potential ideas for presentations, no matter what method you use to gather them. If you're more of an extrovert and you think as you talk, you may like speaking your ideas into a tape recorder. Then you can empty your ideas into a list on a computer file that you print out and paste periodically into your notebook. If you're more of an introvert, you may prefer to write your ideas into a pocket-sized notebook that you keep with you. Or you may want to write the ideas that pop up throughout the day on Post-Its that you arrange in your notebook each evening. Once you figure out what supplies you'll need to keep track of your ideas, you'll have the perfect assignment and destination for your next artist's date.

Jot Box 19-2

Supplies needed:

_____

_____

_____

Destination:

_____

_____

_____

Artist's date & time:

_____

_____

_____

Think presentation and the problems that used to bug you will be transformed into challenges or visions of the possible that are intriguing enough to develop into a presentation.

TIP

Collecting ideas for presentations is like catching butterflies; they are easier to catch when you've got a proper net.

What's Your Idea's Glitter Score?

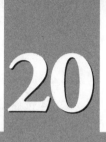

*Always leave enough time in your life
to do something that makes you
happy, satisfied, even joyous.*

Paul Hawken

Now that you've got a way to cull your ideas from everyday experiences, how do you tell which one is intriguing enough to turn into a presentation? There are two ways. Whichever one you choose, your goal is to end up with a single idea that makes your eyes glitter. The first method is to *go for the glitter!* To find an idea for your presentation that's so eye-glittering[1] that it leaves you breathless, write your challenge(s) from Jot Box 19-1 in Jot Box 20-1.

Jot Box 20-1

My Challenge(s)

A. _____

B. _____

C. _____

Now place your three challenges on the following continuum according to their eye-glitter score.

Least Glitter			Moderate Glitter				Most Glitter		
0	1	2	3	4	5	6	7	8	9	10

The Eye-Glitter Scale

Where did you place your challenges along your continuum? Were there any surprises? Because this is the idea you're committing to turning into a presentation, take the time to find a challenge with a glitter-score close to 10. Personally, I won't pursue presentation ideas that score below a 9. If you put an idea on the continuum only to realize that the idea never had much glitter in the first place or that it's lost glitter over time, it's time to search for a new idea.

The second method to determine an idea's glitter score is to *ask a colleague or two* to listen as you tell them about each challenge. They'll be able to tell you which idea makes your voice sparkle or your eyes glitter. If you're one of those lucky people with ideas oozing from your pores, this strategy is particularly useful in picking a single idea with the highest glitter score.

How does the glitter score apply when you've been assigned an unappealing or unfamiliar topic? Say you've been tapped to give a command performance at grand rounds or you're a staff development educator with a critical care background that never prepared you to present on sepsis to a group of maternity nurses. Gifted presenters can and do find the glitter in any topic. You'll learn how to make this happen in Chapter 28 when we talk about slants.

So whether you've chosen or been assigned a topic, it's commitment time. Write the single idea you want to, or have to, turn into a presentation in Jot Box 20-2.

Jot Box 20-2

Your eye-glittering idea is . . .

_____

_____

_____

_____

_____

Great presentations are shaped around a single idea. The more passionate you are about your idea, the easier it is design a presentation that beguiles your audience participants.

TIP

The higher the glitter score, the more fun it is to turn your challenge into an idea for a presentation.

References

1. Hedin, D. (1989, July–August). With eyes a'glitter: Journey to the curriculum revolution. *Nurse Educator, 14*(4), 3–5.

What's a Presentation Worksheet?

21

*Learn the rules so you know
how to break them properly.*

H. Jackson Brown

Every time I break my own rule I kick myself. Someone calls and asks me to present to his or her group. When I pull out a yellow pad and start scribbling without first organizing the project, I get more frantic as minutes turn into hours and I'm still no closer to delivering on my promise to come up with a presentation. When I back up and break down the project into small steps, the fog lifts, the path is clear, and what seemed overwhelming is now doable. It's the difference between hiking a mountain trail one step at a time or standing at the base without a map wondering how you'll get to the top.

During her writing for a publication workshop, Suzanne Hall Johnson[1] introduced me to the four essentials that have served as a compass for my publishing career—idea, slant, audience, and vehicle. As it turns out, these four essentials are as useful for presentations as they are for publications. The Presentation Worksheet introduced in this section expands upon these original four to include all you need to know to design your own presentation.

Presentation Worksheet
Idea: _____
Topic: _____
Focus: _____
Purpose: _____
Audience: _____
Venue: _____
Desired audience response: _____
Slant: _____
One-sentence description: _____

Three examples of actual presentations—shoe-buying when diabetic, nurses caring for themselves, and promoting good hygiene for fifth graders—will be used in this section to show you how to address each item on the worksheet. In the process, you'll complete your first worksheet. Complete a Presentation Worksheet every time you initiate a presentation project and you've got yourself a powerful practice not to mention a versatile tool. You can change the sequence and add and subtract items to ensure that your Presentation Worksheet fits your needs and the requirements of any project.

TIP

Complete your worksheet step-by-step and before you know it you'll have all that you need to design a presentation.

References

1. Johnson, S. H. (1979). *Publishing workshop*. Lakewood, CO: Health Update.

How to Whittle Your Idea to a Presentation-Size Focus

22

A moment's insight is sometimes worth a life's experience.

Oliver Wendell Holmes

Once you identify an eye-glittering idea, there's no end to the presentations you can create. Although an idea is a great place to begin, it's easy to get overwhelmed by the possibilities. To show you how to whittle your eye-glittering idea to a presentation-sized focus, let's start with the shoe-buying when diabetic example because it's so easy to understand.[1] Notice how a general *idea* gets whittled down to a more specific *topic* to an even more specific *focus* in this worksheet.

Presentation Worksheet
Idea: Diabetes
Topic: Diabetic Foot Care
Focus: What people with diabetes should focus on when purchasing new shoes.

Diabetes, as a general *idea,* could take a presentation in a zillion directions. The *topic* zones in on a specific aspect of this big idea—diabetic foot care. The *focus* narrows the idea to a single challenge—what people with diabetes should focus on when purchasing new shoes. Isn't it easier to imagine designing a presentation around purchasing new shoes than around diabetes?

One of the challenges that makes my eyes glitter is helping nurses care for themselves, so the second presentation example is one of my own:

Presentation Worksheet

Idea: Caring for the Caregiver

Topic: Nurses Nurturing Themselves

Focus: Ways for nurses to take better care of themselves so they can care better for others.

The general *idea* is related to caregivers, the *topic* specifies nurses, and the *focus* narrows the challenge to nurses caring for themselves so they can care for others.

Remember Ann's free-write about her middle-school kids' hygiene? Hers is the third example, and you'll see how her free-write challenge translates into the idea/topic/focus strategy.

Ann's Free-Write

I work with middle-school children. I can tell when fifth graders are having trouble keeping up with the changes in their bodies because their hygiene suffers. It's embarrassing for us both when a kid comes into my office and I notice an odor that shouldn't be there or when they get referred by a teacher with a request that I speak to them about cleaning up their act. I want to develop a humorous, interactive presentation on good hygiene that can be given to all the fifth grade classes and repeated yearly with new classes.

Presentation Worksheet

Idea: Hygiene

Topic: Good Hygiene Practices for Fifth Graders

Focus: What fifth graders need to know about good hygiene.

Stated in the most general terms, Ann's *idea* is hygiene. Ann's *topic* specifies a group—fifth graders. Ann's *focus* narrows the idea to reflect the challenge identified in her free-write—what fifth graders need to know about good hygiene.

Are you getting the hang of this? Good, because it's your turn to identify an idea, a topic, and a focus related to your eye-glittering challenge (Jot Box 22-1).

Jot Box 22-1

Your eye-glittering challenge:

_____

_____

Idea:

_____

_____

Topic:

_____

_____

Focus:

_____

_____

Don't turn to the next chapter until you're satisfied that you've whittled your idea to a focused topic. Reread your responses to make sure that your *idea* is stated in the most general terms, that your *topic* is more specific, and that your *focus* narrows your idea to presentation size.

> **TIP**
>
> Shape your presentation around a single, eye-glittering idea whittled down to a focused topic.

References

1. Heinrich, K. T., Neese, R., Rogers, D., & Facente, A. (2004, May–June). Turning accusations into affirmations: Transform nurses into published authors. *Nursing Education Perspectives, 25*(2), 139–145.

Present What You Do
Strategies and Skills

What's Your Purpose?

Learn to get in touch with the silence within yourself, and know that everything in this life has purpose. There are no mistakes, no coincidences, all events are blessings given to us to learn from.

Elisabeth Kubler-Ross

When Beverly Sastri,[1] a colleague–friend in my support circle, got the opportunity to speak about her CD describing her work at our local bookstore, she asked me to be her peer mentor. We spent several hours debating the advantages and disadvantages of various presentation designs. During our debriefing session after her presentation, Beverly said she was disappointed in her CD sales following her presentation. As we spoke, we figured out why she hadn't sold more CDs. Although her purpose for giving the presentation was to sell CDs, Beverly never showed the audience what the CD looked like or mentioned what they would get from listening to it. Although we both knew that selling CDs was her purpose, we ignored it when it came to designing her presentation. Lesson learned. It's important to keep your purpose front and center as you design your presentations.

77

The purpose of a presentation may include one or more of the following:

1. To educate
2. To motivate, awaken, alert, agitate
3. To design or advertise a product
4. To gain professional recognition
5. To get personal satisfaction
6. To garner institutional visibility

In the shoe-buying when diabetic example, the purpose is educating the public:

Presentation Worksheet

Idea: Diabetes

   Topic: Diabetic Foot Care

   Focus: What people with diabetes should focus on when purchasing new shoes.

Purpose: *Educate.* To raise a lay audience's awareness and offer
suggestions about proper footwear for those with diabetes.

As you can see, specifying your purpose helps to determine the presentation's content.

In my "nurses nurturing themselves" presentation, the purpose is to motivate nursing audiences to care for themselves. Note that I borrowed the phrasing from the diabetic example to frame the purpose for my presentation:

Presentation Worksheet

Idea: Caring for the Caregiver

Topic: Nurses Nurturing Themselves

Focus: Ways for nurses to take better care of themselves so they can care better for others.

Purpose: *Motivate*. To raise nurses' awareness and offer suggestions for self-nurturing strategies so they can care for others without neglecting their own needs.

By contrast, Ann's presentation has three purposes, one related to what will be presented, another related to how it will be presented, and a third related to how often:

Presentation Worksheet

Idea: Hygiene

Topic: Good Hygiene Practices for Fifth Graders

Focus: What fifth graders need to know about good hygiene.

Purpose:

1. *Educate*. Raise fifth grader's awareness about good hygiene.

2. *Motivate*. Offer suggestions for products that make for good hygiene.

3. *Design Product*. Develop a humorous, interactive presentation that's repeatable.

Now that you've seen the purpose for each example, what's the purpose for your presentation? Feel free to use the sentence structure from any of the examples above to formulate your statement of purpose (Jot Box 23-1).

Jot Box 23-1

Idea: _____

_____

Topic: _____

Focus: _____

Purpose: _____

_____

As you'll see, identifying your purpose helps clarify decisions as you design your presentation. Not only that, when you're writing a proposal that asks for your purpose, you'll have a well-considered response.

TIP

Keep your purpose "front-stage" to design a presentation to meet that purpose.

References

1. Sastri, B. (2004). *Create a life you love* [CD]. Self-published.

Who's Your Audience?

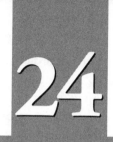

*When I'm talking to a large audience, I imagine
that I'm talking to a single person.*

Red Barber

When it comes to audiences, size matters. So does the composition of
the audience you're addressing—lay or professional; children, adoles-
cents, young adults, middle-aged adults, or elders; and/or special characteristics shared, such as a particular concern or diagnosis. By taking
audience size and composition into consideration, we'll see what's
known about the audience in our three examples.

The audience for the shoe-buying when diabetic presentation is as
follows:

Audience: Lay public; 100 to 150 people who have diabetes or
who have a family member with diabetes.

The number of audience participants influences not only what you
present but how you present. With an audience of 100 to 150 lay people, for example, what's the best way for them to introduce themselves
to each other? You might ask them to turn to the person sitting behind
them and introduce themselves. As far as composition, this is a lay audience, so you'll need to make decisions about whether to use professional
jargon or terms your great-grandmother would understand.

In the case of the presentation on nurses nurturing themselves:

Audience: Professional audience; 200 nurses from across specialties in Connecticut.

With professional audiences, it's important to know which disciplines or specialty areas you're addressing. Over the years, I've shared this presentation with hospice nurses, community health nurses, hospital-based nurses, and students enrolled in nursing programs ranging from LPN to doctoral. In each case, my audience determined the examples I used. Because this audience is a mixed group of nurses from across Connecticut, I can use examples from a range of settings familiar to those living in our state.

In the final example, Ann's audience is also a lay audience:

Audience: Fifth graders—three classes with 25 to 29 children in each class.

When it comes to presenting to an audience of children, Ann needs to consider their developmental life stage. Although Ann sees these students in her health office, asking teachers what they see in the classroom may enable her to better address students' learning needs around hygiene in an age-appropriate manner.

What you don't know can be more important than what you know about your audience. Take the shoe-buying when diabetic presentation, for instance. In addition to not knowing the exact number of audience members, you may not know whether they are newly diagnosed. If knowing this would help you design your presentation, there are three options:

1. *Ask.* Contact someone who knows or who knows somebody who knows.
2. *Assess learning needs.* Contact audience members beforehand to conduct what adult educators call a "learning needs assessment." E-mail allows for presession assessments that include brief surveys or open-ended questions such as, "What would you like to learn from this presentation?" Their responses give you a good idea about the issues your audience would like to see addressed.
3. *Prepare several versions of the presentation.* Offer audiences a couple of options and ask them to choose. For example, Beverly has a lecture version and an interactive version of her intro-

ductory presentation. Note that this third option is possible only when you're comfortable with the content and expert enough to be flexible in your presentation design.

When you describe your audience in Jot Box 24-1, be as specific as possible.

Jot Box

1. How many people will be in the audience?

_____

2. What is the composition of your audience?

_____

3. What do you know about your audience?

_____

4. What do you need to find out about your audience?

_____

Find out the answers to these four questions during the planning process to design a presentation that fits your audience participants to a tee.

TIP
The more you know about the size and composition of your audience-participants, the better.

How to Choreograph Your Venue

25

> *I was 58 years old when I finally felt like a "master choreographer." . . . for the first time in my life I felt in control of all the components that go into making a dance—the music, the steps, the patterns, the deployment of people onstage, the clarity of purpose. Finally I had the skills to close the gap between what I could see in my mind and what I could actually get onto the stage.*
>
> Twyla Tharp

The *venue* is the physical setting where the presentation happens. In retrospect, some of my most unpleasant presenting experiences have been the result of an audience–venue mismatch. The times when I've facilitated a workshop for 6 people in a cavernous hotel ballroom with seating for 2,000, brought 25 handouts to find the room packed with 75 overheated people squished into a room that seats 35, or tried to engage audiences in small-group exercises when they're seated face-forward, auditorium style.

These experiences have taught me to anticipate such choreographic challenges by gathering as much information as possible about the venue beforehand. To get your choreographic career off to a good start, check out the fit between audience and venue in each of our three examples:

Presentation Worksheet

Audience: Lay public; 100 to 150 people who have diabetes or who have a family member with diabetes

Venue: Community hospital cafeteria that seats up to 200 people

Choreographic challenges: Seating arrangements, acoustics, and external noise level

---

For the number of people expected—between 100 and 150—the seating is more than adequate. That said, a venue like a cafeteria comes with significant choreographic challenges. Cafeterias are designed for eating, not presenting; people are seated at large round or long tables. Not only is it difficult to hear, you can find yourself yelling over the noise of dishes crashing in the kitchen.

In the case of the nurses caring for themselves presentation example:

Presentation Worksheet

Audience: Professional audience; 200 nurses from across specialties

Venue: An auditorium that seats 300 people

Choreographic challenges: Stationary seating arrangements

In this example, there's a good fit between the size of the audience and the venue. Although most auditoriums have adequate acoustics and external noise control, the challenge here is choreographing interactive exercises. Sometimes, for example, I'll ask every set of two people to turn around to face the two people behind them so the entire audience ends up divided into foursomes for small-group experiences.

In Ann's case:

Presentation Worksheet
Audience: Fifth graders; three classes with between 25 and 29 children in each class and their teachers
Venue: A rectangular, all-purpose room with a stage at the front overlooking a large expanse of linoleum floor with folding chairs stored in heaps against the back wall. This space accommodates up to 250 people.
Choreographic challenges: Best place for presenter to stand to be seen

Because Ann's audience involves three fifth-grade classes, she knows the size and the composition of her audience. From having already presented in this room, Ann also knows that the kids sit on the linoleum floor in a couple of loose, concentric circles, with teachers standing or seated on folding chairs behind the kids. Ann plans to keep her audience-participants' attention by standing on the stage where she can see and be seen.

Whether you're familiar with your venue or not, the best way to anticipate choreographic challenges is to answer the following questions. Feel free to add your own questions to this list.

1. What is the room used for (e.g. classroom, seminar, cafeteria, auditorium)?
2. What is the seating arrangement? Stationary? Moveable?
3. What is the lighting (e.g. natural light from windows, overhead fluorescent, etc.)?
4. How private is this room? Are there any competing presentations in same room?

5. What are the acoustics like?
6. How well insulated is the room for temperature? For blocking out external sounds?
7. What is the fit between the size of your audience and the presentation room?
8. How will this room fit your presentation style? Your purpose? Your audience?
9. What type of audiovisual equipment is available?
10. What obstructions, such as columns, may prevent speakers from seeing and being seen?

Consider the following basic operating principle: If you create an ambience that makes you comfortable, your audience-participants will feel comfortable as well. Even when you don't know and can't find out where you're presenting, as is the case when conferences are held at hotels and conference centers, it's safe to anticipate two choreographic challenges: seating and beautification. With regard to seating, always get to your venue 30 to 45 minutes early. Depending on the size of the audience, arrange seats in a circle or a herringbone configuration, as opposed to rows, so participants can see each other.

To make venues as aesthetically appealing as possible, I bring the following three items to every presentation:

- A CD with a mix of soothing songs
- A CD player
- A vase of flowers or a flowering plant

The first thing I do is turn on my CD player. The soft instrumental music calms me and creates a soothing environment for participants as they arrive. While arranging the seating for group activities, I place a yellow dot under the seat of a chair. Whoever finds the dot under their seat "wins" the flowers. If I have a say in the matter, my presentation packet covers are colorful. I encourage conveners to provide healthy snacks, because sugary snacks raise and drop glucose levels precipitously, leaving participants drowsy.

Now it's time to write what is known about your venue in Jot Box 25-1.

Jot Box 25-1
---

1. What do you know about your venue?

_____

_____

_____

_____

2. What do you need to know about your venue?

_____

_____

_____

_____

3. What are your choreographic challenges?

_____

_____

_____

_____

Compromise is as important as choreography in fitting venue to audience, because most venues have at least one choreographic challenge that can and one that can't be anticipated.

TIP

The more you anticipate choreographic challenges, the freer you'll be to meet the unanticipated ones.

What Response Are You Seeking from Your Audience?

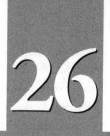

Your audience gives you everything you need. They tell you. There is no director who can direct you like an audience.

Fanny Brice

I was asked to be the after-lunch speaker for 165 health-care administrators and staff nurses from across the state. The venue was a cafeteria with 20 round tables that each seated 8 people. Because this was a yearly event for people who didn't get to see each other during the year, the decibel level during lunch was deafening. The audience kept talking over the convener as she introduced me, so I was relieved to see that they quieted down once I took the podium. Had I given a lecture, they might have stayed quiet. But noooo, I had to go interactive. After giving them a minute to dialogue about a question with the person next to them, I tried my best to bring them back. They just kept chattering away. At the end of the longest half hour of my life, I sat down red-faced and took the earliest opportunity to scuttle out the backdoor.

Until that audience's response ran so counter to my *unexpressed expectations*, I'd never given much thought to the response I expect from my audience. Based on this insight, I added an item called the "desired audience response" to the Presentation Worksheet. Table 26-1 links the presentation purpose with the desired audience response.

TABLE 26-1   Purpose and Desired Audience Response for Presentations

---

Purpose	Desired Audience Response
Educate	Learn
Motivate	Inspire/move to action
Design/advertise product	Buy product
Professional recognition	Promotion, tenure, etc.
Personal satisfaction	Appreciation, gratitude
Institutional visibility	Article in the press, etc.

Let's see how purpose relates to audience response in each of our three examples. In the shoe-buying when diabetic presentation:

Presentation Worksheet

Purpose: *Educate*. To raise a lay audience's awareness and offer suggestions about proper footwear for those with diabetes

Desired audience response: After this presentation, participants will know what to consider when buying shoes for someone with diabetes.

When the purpose is *education*, the desired audience response involves *learning*.

In the case of nurses taking care of themselves:

Presentation Worksheet

Purpose: *Motivate*. To raise nurses' awareness of the need for self-nurturing strategies so they can care for others without neglecting their own needs

Desired audience response: After this presentation, participants will commit to one self-nurturing strategy to complete in the next week.

Because the purpose is to *motivate*, the desired audience response is to *inspire* and *move to action*.

In Ann's example, there are two desired responses: an increase in awareness and use of hygiene products.

Presentation Worksheet

Purpose:

1. *Educate*—raise fifth grader's awareness about good hygiene.

2. *Motivate*—offer suggestions for products that make for good hygiene.

Desired audience response: Exhibit improved hygiene resulting from the proper use of hygiene products.

In this final example, where the purpose is both to *educate* and to *motivate*, the desired audience response is to *move to action* as a result of *learning*.

Note that in all three examples, the desired audience responses relate to action inspired by learning and motivation. By framing audience responses in action-oriented and learner-centered terms, you're writing what educators call *behavioral objectives*.[1] It's your turn to decide on the desired audience response for your presentation (Jot Box 26-1). Don't forget to use Table 26-1 to match your desired audience response to your purpose.

Jot Box 26-1

Your purpose:

_____

_____

Your desired audience response:

_____

_____

_____

Did it work? By anticipating a desired audience response during the design phase, you've increased the probability that your presentation will elicit that response. Beyond this assessment measure of desired audience response, you've just identified a behavioral objective written in action-oriented and learner-centered language.

Now we're going to make a leap that might surprise you. Although it's common wisdom to get an idea and search the literature, in her publishing workshop, Suzanne Hall Johnson encouraged us to wait until we clarified our own ideas. That way, you're much less likely to lose your own idea in the sea of ideas washing over you as you search the literature. Now that you've clarified your idea, this is the perfect time for a literature search.

Pam Walker, a nurse educator and creative writer, is so skilled at searching the literature that I've asked her to walk you through the steps of conducting a literature search in Chapter 27.

TIP
By anticipating a desired audience response, you can measure how closely their actual response matches the response you'd hoped for.

References

1. Bastable, S. B. (2000). *Nurse as educator: Principles of teaching and learning for nursing practice* (2nd ed.). Sudbury, MA: Jones and Bartlett.

How to Take the Dare Out of Your Literature Search

27

Pam Walker, RN, MSN

If you're going to do a thing,
you should do it thoroughly.

Muriel Sparks

I suspect that those of you with limited experience are facing the challenge of searching the literature with trepidation. Fear not! As nurses, you've been trained in the fine art of interviewing patients and gathering physical data. Now you can turn your natural detective instincts toward searching the literature for abstracts, articles, and books that carry the most up-to-date thinking on your focused topic. When preparing presentations, a literature search can provide you with the most recent, cutting-edge information that will "wow" your audience. In the case of a journal article, be it informal or scholarly, the key is to discover what has already been written and published so you can slant your topic in a way that's intriguing and publishable (see Section 3). Using Kathy's example of the "nurses nurturing themselves" presentation example, this chapter walks you step-by-step through the process of searching the literature.

Step 1. Identify Key Words

The first step is identifying those words that best describe and are most closely related to your focused topic. Using Kathy's presentation topic, key words would include "nurses," "stress," "nurturing," "caring," etc. Take a

93

minute or two and use Jot Box 27-1 to list key words or concepts that apply to your focused topic.

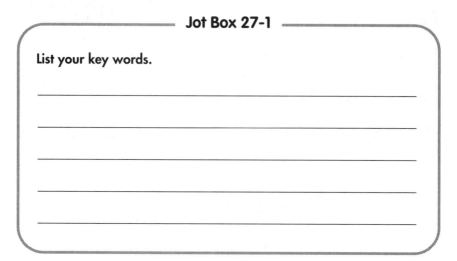

Jot Box 27-1

List your key words.

Step 2. Translate Key Words into Synonyms

Review your list, cluster your key words or concepts, make a list of synonyms, and combine terms for greater specificity using Kathy's presentation example as a guide (Information Box 27-1).

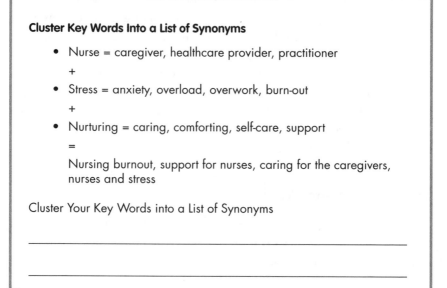

Information Box 27-1

Cluster Key Words Into a List of Synonyms

- Nurse = caregiver, healthcare provider, practitioner
  +
- Stress = anxiety, overload, overwork, burn-out
  +
- Nurturing = caring, comforting, self-care, support
  =

  Nursing burnout, support for nurses, caring for the caregivers, nurses and stress

Cluster Your Key Words into a List of Synonyms

With that task completed, you're ready to start your search!

Step 3. Define Your Terms

Whenever nurses are faced with conducting a literature search, they ask the three questions discussed here.

Question 1: What is a literature search?

The literature search "tells both what is known and not known about a particular topic" (p. 1).[1] Searching the literature familiarizes you with what's out there, what's not out there, and how you can fill the gap. It provides your audience with the most up-to-date information on practice issues and lends authenticity to your presentation.

Question 2: Why do a literature search?

It's a good idea to do a literature search whether you're writing about your practice or describing a research project. When they hear the term *literature search*, many nurses think "research" and scare themselves. The "R" word—research can call out nurses' impostor syndrome big-time. They think if they don't do research, they get to skip the literature search step. Even if your goal is not a scholarly research project, the literature search keeps you focused on your specific topic and prevents duplication of others' work. And, who knows? Maybe your detective work will inspire a new avenue of interest that makes your eyes glitter and result in other presentations or publications.

Question 3: What's the difference between a literature search and a literature review?

It's important to avoid confusing the term *literature search* with *literature review*. In the language of the nursing process, think of the literature search as the "assessment" phase of the nursing process, the gathering of data, the detective work. The literature review is the "planning" step when we take that data, analyze what it means, and select and synthesize the most pertinent informational points to present or publish.[1]

Now that we've clarified definitions and terms, it's time to talk about the steps involved in conducting a literature search.

Step 4. Begin Your Search

To those of us of a certain age who cringe at the words "Readers' Guide to Periodical Literature," I say, "Welcome to the age of electronic databases!" You have a choice. Go to the library and get guidance on conducting a computer search or do your search from home on your computer. You may be affiliated with a college or university or have a kind friend who works at a facility with a substantial medical and/or nursing library. If not, there is probably a library nearby that, for a small fee, will allow you to search their electronic databases, one of which may well be the online version of the Readers' Guide! Most libraries subscribe to database services such as EBSCOhost that provide you with access to multiple databases. For information on nursing and related practice, visit the valuable databases listed in Information Box 27-2.

Information Box 27-2

Valuable Databases

- CINAHL (Cumulative Index to Nursing and Allied Health Literature)
- Academic Search Elite
- ERIC (Educational research database)
- PsychInfo (American Psychological Association)
- MEDLINE.gov (U.S. National Library of Medicine)

The website of the National Library of Medicine, www.nlm.nih.gov, is also an excellent source of free literature and other educational products.

Additional sources for recent articles are the websites of nursing magazines and journals, such as *Nursing Education Perspectives* at www.nln.org/nlnjournal or *RN Magazine* at www.rnweb.com and nursing specialty societies like the Oncology Nursing Society at www.ons.org or the American Nurses Association website, www.nursingworld.org. Often these sites will have links to archived articles, those published in previous editions of a journal, many for free or a minimal processing charge.

Finally, you can go directly to the Internet and research your topic using a search engine such as www.google.com, www.ask.com, www.yahoo.com, etc. Remember, however, that no one polices the accuracy of information on the Internet. My advice is to trust *only* the information on reputable, verifiable sites, such as those affiliated with recognized healthcare organizations or government agencies.

Step 5. Conduct Your Search

Right now you're sitting in front of your computer screen looking at the search engine or database you've chosen, asking yourself, "Now what? Can I really do this?" Just relax and simply type your key word(s) in the space labeled "search," click "submit" or "go" and you're off and running. In the databases, you can refine your search by selecting specific years or limiting the search to only full-text articles, so that the entire article can be viewed online. Your search will result in a list, beginning with the most recent, of all articles that contain those key words in their titles. Often, you'll need to further refine your key word search if you wish to eliminate articles which may not apply to nursing.

For example, using my cluster list, I typed "nurses and stress" into my database. The result was a list of more than 7000 articles that contained those two key words. A quick scan of the first 20 to 30 "hits" told me that I needed a more refined search. "Nursing burnout" narrowed the search down to only three articles. Obviously, I needed to find a happy medium! That's what your search of the literature will be—trial and error, joy and disappointment. The trick is to stay focused on the topic at hand and not be tempted, as I often am, to take an interesting side trip down another road.

Next, click on the title of an article that applies to your focused topic. You will find an abstract, or description, of the article content and a link to a full-text document if available.

Step 6. Expand Your Search

Most databases offer full-text versions of many of their articles. When the entire article is available to be viewed online, you can print it out or download and save it to your computer's hard drive. This is a wonderful timesaver, as you can quickly scan these articles to make sure they are appropriate for your search and then save them or reject them and move on! However, if the entire article you want is not available for download, you will need to take your search a step further. Make a list of those articles, including the journal name, year, and volume number. Then take that list and search the electronic "card catalogue" on the nearest college or university website to see if they have the journals you're looking for. If they do, a trip to the library and a pocketful of dimes, nickels, or quarters for the copier are all you'll need to complete your search. Remember to be aware of copyright laws and any specific library restrictions regarding photocopying.

Step 7. Search for Gaps, Slants, and New Leads

So, you've searched the literature, you've identified the abstracts and articles that you're interested in, and you've tracked them down. Now it's time to find yourself a quiet place to review all the leads that your detective work turned up. Don't forget to check the reference list at the end of each article. You can get additional information by reviewing the authors' source materials as well. Again, it's a fine balance between being open to new thinking and staying true to the focused topic that you chose before you reviewed the literature.

As you look through your sources, keep an eye out for the gaps in what's been written—what's been covered well and what hasn't been thoroughly addressed. These gaps help you to identify potential slants which are unique takes on your focused topic. Slants are covered in more detail in the next chapter.

Conclusion

Your presentations and publications will be more persuasive when you cite sources that are up-to-the-minute. To recap, your literature search is one part information gathering, one part detective work, and infinite parts exciting journey. Just remember, this is really nothing new: Whatever your practice, you've been doing "information searches" for years! Get ready to return to your Presentation Worksheet to identify a snappy slant informed by your review of the literature.

TIP
Beware of the tempting adventure down the side road. Stay on course!

References

1. Heinrich, K. T. (2002, Winter). Slant, style, and synthesis: 3 keys to a strong literature review. *Nurse Author & Editor: A Newsletter for Nurse Authors, Reviewers and Editors, 12*(1), 1–3.

How to Snag a Sweet-Spot Slant

28

I can't recall the last time I wasn't on the hunt for a good title. Titles are crucial. Titles can give a literary work a frame or a spark. They can infuse a piece with power and authority, or with mystery and allure. Thomas Lux, a poet, says that a poet's job is to write poems that are hard not to read. A title sets up that inevitability. This title stakes a claim. It immediately reaches out and grasps the reader's imagination.

Van Wickel

How do you decide which magazine to buy for that long plane flight? The same way you decide which presentation to attend at a professional conference. It's a headline that grabs your attention; a title that's relevant to your life. A slant is a fresh and unique perspective on a topic. Titles with irresistible slants make it hard not to buy a particular magazine or attend a particular conference session. Now that you've narrowed your eye-glittering idea to a focused topic, named your purpose, identified your audience, described your venue, and considered a desirable audience response, you have enough information to craft your slant. I say *craft,* because when you're in the market for sexy slants playfulness and creativity come in handy.

Titles can be descriptive, emotive, or a combination of both. Descriptive (D) titles tell the reader exactly what the book is about; emotive (E) titles grab you by the heart and won't let go. Take the title of this book for example. As you can see from the eye-glitter scores below, the three titles on my original short list were all Ds. Because not a one contained an E phrase, they were also lackluster:

Three Potential Titles and Eye-Glitter Scores

Share What You Do: Presenting & Publishing Made Easy For Nurses	7
Nurses: Present and Publish What You Do	7
Just Share What You Do: The Easy Way for Nurses to Present and Publish	5

After Christina Purpora, a nurse colleague, agreed to serve as a peer editor, we were playing with different slants when the phrase "dare to share" popped out of my mouth. It was like hearing the ping of a baseball hitting the sweet spot on a bat. A 10 on the eye-glitter continuum, we knew right then and there that "dare to share" had to be part of the title. That made the final title a combination of a D and an E. *A Nurse's Guide to Presenting and Publishing* is the descriptive phrase; *Dare to Share* is the sweet-spot slant that makes it hard for potential readers to pass this book by without taking a peek.

See how sweet spot slants in our three presentation examples become titles that match message to audience. In the diabetes example:

Presentation Worksheet

Slant (Title): When Buying New Shoes (D), What You Don't Know Can Hurt You (E)

This twist in the E title would tantalize a lay audience by suggesting that no matter what they know about diabetes, there's more to learn about buying shoes.

If nailing a slant looks easy, don't be fooled! Good slants can take time and tweaking to develop. Because I've facilitated presentations on nurses nurturing themselves over the years for many different audiences, I've played with a lot of different slants and titles. For me, the most sweet-spot slant ended up being:

Presentation Worksheet
Slant (Title): Come to Your Senses: The Gentle Art of Nurturing Yourself

The phrase, "come to your senses," came from a series of articles in the *Utne Reader*,[1] a periodical I read regularly because it's a reliable source of the latest social trends. Trends inspire slants that are engaging because they are timely. As you read newspapers, periodicals, and books published in the popular press, be on the lookout for trends that lend themselves to slants for your own presentations.

Ann listed a descriptive title and a couple of options that she's playing with for her sweet-spot title. She's been asking teachers, other school nurses, parents, and kids to help her find a snappy title (which, by the way, is a great way to track down a sweet-spot slant). Of the three listed, which E title grabs you the most?

- It's Cool!: Look Good, Smell Great
- Look Good, Smell Great: How to Make It Happen
- Hygiene Is Not a Dirty Word

If you want your presentation to stand out from the rest, don't stop until you hear the ping that sweet-spot slants make. Your challenge is to make your titles so descriptive *and* engaging that participants can't wait to attend your presentation. Because it's often easier to start out with a descriptive title, I've given you room to write both a D and an E title in Jot Box 28-1. Remember that the most powerful titles are combinations of D and E titles.

Jot Box 28-1

Your D title: _____

+

Your E title: _____

Play with the order of your titles—D + E or E + D—until you find the best sounding, most attractive combination.

Many nurses stop at descriptive titles. To enthrall audience participants, your title must go beyond the descriptive and call their hearts to sing, sigh, or sob. There is no more powerful combination!

TIP

If an idea was a pie, the slant would be the juiciest, plumpest piece chosen to delight your audience participants' taste buds.

References

1. Olson, K. (2001, November/December). Tasting the wind, hearing the water. In Born sensuous: How to recharge your batteries by coming back to your senses. *Utne Reader: The Best of Alternative Press.* No. 108.

How to Complete Your Presentation Worksheet

29

I don't wait for moods. You accomplish nothing if you do that. Your mind must know it has got to get down to earth.

Pearl S. Buck

A couple of months ago I received the following e-mail message from Dr. Judy Farnsworth, a nurse educator and colleague–friend:

> Just wanted you to know how helpful your focusing worksheet has been. I spent a couple of hours Sunday helping a student who is working on her thesis. She had grand ideas for her project: too many, too varied, too flakey. I copied that sheet. Had her sit down and do it! And BINGO! We could finally move on to more nuts and bolts.

Even though it takes concentration and creative energy to complete a Presentation Worksheet, doing so saves you untold time and aggravation by ensuring that your presentation's conceptual design is airtight from the get-go.

You, too, can have that same bingo experience by transfering the items that you've written into your Jot Boxes in the last 10 chapters onto the "Presentation Worksheet" on page 106. You may notice that these items look different when listed on a single page. Some that seemed fine as separate ideas don't hang together. One of the best things about the Presentation Worksheet is that it sheds light on the holes or discrepancies in your thinking. Notice that the shoe-buying when diabetic presentation worksheet serves as an example to make sure that each item flows logically from the item before.

When you complete your own worksheet, leave the item "One-sentence description" blank; we'll work through that together in Chapter 30.

Presentation Worksheet

Idea: Diabetes

Topic: Diabetic foot care

Focus: What those with diabetes should focus on when purchasing new shoes.

Purpose: To raise awareness among the lay public about the smart way to buy shoes when they or a loved one have diabetes

Audience: Lay public; 100 to 150 people

Venue: Wellness presentation in community hospital conference room; seats up to 200 people

Desired audience response: After this presentation, participants know what to consider when buying shoes for someone with diabetes.

Slant (Title): When buying new shoes, what you don't know *can* hurt you.

One-sentence description:

Your Presentation Worksheet

Idea: _____

_____

Topic: _____

Focus: _____

Purpose: _____

Audience: _____

Venue: _____

Desired audience response: _____

Slant: _____

One-sentence description: Stay tuned and we'll complete this item in Chapter 30.

Are your worksheet items as on target as those in the diabetes example? To find out, answer the following questions:

1. Does your venue fit your audience?
2. Does your purpose fit your desired audience response?
3. Does the slant include both a descriptive and an emotive component?

When you answer yes to all three questions, the items listed on your Presentation Worksheet flow logically from one to another.

Now you're ready for the final step in completing this worksheet—composing a one-sentence description.

TIP

Complete a Worksheet to make sure that your presentation centers around a single idea that is logically developed.

How to Write Your One-Sentence Description

30

*Creative minds have always been known
to survive any bad training.*

Anna Freud

The final step in completing your Worksheet is formulating a single sentence that describes your presentation. When you can do this, you know what you want to present. Our three examples show what good descriptive sentences look like. Let's start with a one-sentence description of the shoe-buying when diabetic presentation. See if you can spot the problem with this one-sentence description:

Presentation Worksheet

One-sentence description: Because peripheral neuropathy is common among people with diabetes, incorrect selection of shoes can cause serious and/or permanent foot injuries. This presentation shows how making smart choices when buying shoes can prevent serious and/or permanent foot injuries for those with diabetes.

If you said this in not one, but two sentences, you're right. That's not all! Because this presentation targets a lay audience, it might include people who have never heard of peripheral neuropathy. So let's pare it down to one sentence framed in lay terms:

Presentation Worksheet
One-sentence description: This presentation shows how making smart choices when buying shoes can prevent serious and/or permanent foot injuries for those with diabetes.

What do you think? This description is a single sentence written in language that everyone can understand. As a final test, does this sentence address the focused topic, purpose, audience, and slant? Yes. Because it addresses the education and motivation of those with diabetes to know what about buying shoes can hurt, this sentence is a keeper.

For my presentation on nurses nurturing themselves, my one-sentence description reads:

Presentation Worksheet
One-sentence description: This interactive presentation helps nurses appreciate the importance of renewing themselves by reawakening to their senses and identifying a sensory-renewing activity for the week.

Note that I've added the word *interactive* to describe the workshop so audience participants know that they'll be playing an active role in their own learning.

Ann's one-sentence description reads:

Presentation Worksheet
One-sentence description: During this interactive presentation, students learn about hygiene products that keep them looking and smelling great all day long.

Remember that Ann wanted to develop a fun and interactive way to present good hygiene practices to fifth graders? Her sentence conveys both the fun and the interactive parts of her message.

Now it's your turn to describe your presentation in a single sentence (Jot Box 30-1).

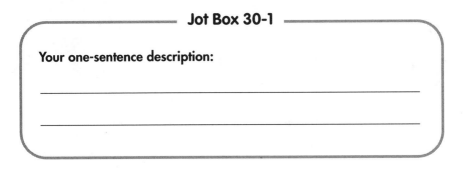

Jot Box 30-1

Your one-sentence description:

_____

_____

Are you satisfied with your one-sentence description? When your sentence addresses your focused topic, purpose, audience, and slant, you're there.

Why not keep a stash of blank Presentation Worksheets handy? Whenever you get an idea, write it on a worksheet and put it in a folder marked "Eye-Glittering Presentation Ideas." Then, when needed, you'll have a bunch of eye-glittering presentation ideas to choose from.

Now that your Presentation Worksheet is complete, you know *what* you want to present. It's time to consider *how* you will present.

TIP

Use your one-sentence description for everything from presentation proposals to session descriptions for conference brochures.

How to Translate Worksheets into Proposals

31

When you've got a dream, you've got to grab it and never let go.

Carol Burnett

When Lisa Nowak, a former student and conference convener, called to ask me to speak at the annual dinner meeting for her school nurse group, we discussed several potential ideas. After our discussion, Lisa asked me to send an e-mail with a list of potential topics. Whether you're responding to a request from a colleague or a formal "Call for Proposals" for a national conference, submitting a proposal is the place to begin. My "proposal" was the following e-mail message.

My Informal Proposal

Dear Lisa:
Brainstorming presentation topics for your group's October 26th Dinner Meeting was fun. Below you'll find the working titles of the three possibilities we discussed for this 50 minute, experiential presentation:

1. Stop the Joy-stealing Games: How to Civilize Relationships with Students, Teachers, Administrators, and Parents
2. With Eye's A'Glitter: Turn Your Passion for School Nursing into Grant Proposals

(continues)

> 3. Come to Your Senses: On the Gentle Art of Nurturing Yourself
>
> Should you require anything further to help you and your committee make your decision, please contact me.
>
> Warmly,
>
> Kathy

I was thrilled to get Lisa's e-mail saying that her committee chose the topic with the highest score on my eye-glitter scale—joy-stealing games. Lisa asked for a session title, description, and a single behavioral objective so they could advertise the session and submit the paperwork for continuing education units (CEUs). It was time to complete a Presentation Worksheet.

My Presentation Worksheet

Idea: Joy-stealing

Topic: Joy-stealing games

Focus: What school nurses need to know about joy-stealing games

Purpose: To educate and awaken school nurses to joy-stealing games and introduce strategies for establishing zestful relationships with students, teachers, administrators, and parents

Audience: 80 to 100 school nurses for the School Nurse Association of Connecticut

Venue: Restaurant Dining Room

(continues)

My Presentation Worksheet (continued)

Desired audience response: To foster zestful school environments with zero-tolerance for such games

Slant (Title): Joy Stealing: What School Nurses Can Do to Stop the Mean Games

One-sentence description: Designed to stimulate spirited dialogue, this interactive session engages participants in sharing stories about situations that stole their joy and strategizing new ways of responding that foster zestful academic environments.

As you can see, deciding on a slant resulted in a session title that combined a descriptive (D) phrase and an emotive (E) phrase. With the worksheet completed, it was easy to compose the session description and the single behavioral objective.

My Proposal

Title: Joy Stealing Games: What School Nurses Can Do to Stop the Game-Playing
Presenter: Kathleen T. Heinrich
Session Description: Designed to stimulate spirited dialogue, this interactive session engages participants in sharing stories about situations with students, teachers, administrators, and parents that steal their joy and strategizing new ways of responding that foster zestful academic environments.
Behavioral Objective: After this workshop, participants will initiate a dialogue about how school nurses can foster zestful school environments with zero-tolerance for joy-stealing games.

Did you notice that the Presentation Worksheet's one-sentence description became the proposal's session description, and the desired audience response became the behavioral objective? Objectives for sessions that offer CEUs must be stated in behavioral terms that begin with the phrase, "After this session, participants will . . ." I make writing objectives in behavioral terms a practice whether or not CEUs are being offered.

Now it's your turn. Whether you've got a gig or you just want the practice, write your own session description and a behavioral objective from your Presentation Worksheet (see page 106).

Jot Box 31-1

Your Proposal

Session Title:

_____

_____

Presenter(s):

_____

_____

Session Description:

_____

_____

_____

_____

Behavioral Objective:

_____

_____

I want to bring two things to your attention. First, informal as our proposal process was, I followed Lisa's guidelines and fulfilled her every request. That's because it's my job as a presenter to make Lisa's job as a convener as easy as possible. Second, seeing how easy it was to translate my worksheet into an informal proposal and trying it yourself may give you a new appreciation for this powerful practice.

After completing the Presentation Worksheet, I knew my greatest challenge was my audience. This was my first time presenting the topic of joy-stealing to a group of school nurses. As you will discover in the next chapter, this insight led me to ask a colleague–friend to act as my peer mentor.

TIP

Get ready! You'll be invited to present when you're recognized as an expert in your field, your topic is hot, or you're known for your signature presenting style.

How to Pick a Peer Mentor

. . . a side-by-side feeling that someone believes in you.

Faith Middleton

Whenever I begin a presentation project, creating a support circle is every bit as important as filling out a Presentation Worksheet. As you can see from the following timeline, I asked Karen Owen to be my peer mentor the second after Lisa said I had the job.

My Timeline for the Joy-Stealing Presentation

Task	Date
1. Phone conversation with Lisa	September 18
2. E-mail presentation options to Lisa	September 25
3. Committee confirms presentation topic	September 25
4. Timeline completed	September 25
5. Karen Owen agrees to be my peer mentor	September 25
6. Presentation Worksheet completed	September 27
7. Joy-Stealing presentation draft completed	September 30
8. Peer-mentoring walk/talk	October 5
9. Peer-mentoring preconference	October 13
10. Presentation	October 26
11. Peer-mentoring postconference	October 26

Once you know more about peer mentoring, you'll understand why reaching out to Karen was anything but a hasty decision and the smartest thing I could have done. The following are the answers to the three most common questions nurses ask about the peer mentoring process:

1. *What is peer mentoring?* Peer mentoring is a scripted feedback model that helps presenters refine their presenting skills over time by reflecting on presentations in the context of a trusting collegial relationship.[1,2] Appreciative rather than evaluative, peer mentoring is unique in that it is presenter driven. This means that presenters ask for the assistance and the type of feedback they need, and peer mentors respect and comply with these requests.

2. *What qualities make for a good peer mentor?* A peer mentor is, above all, a good listener who asks questions and explores inconsistencies. The best peer mentors bring a beginner's mind to presentation topics and question assumptions presenter(s) may take for granted.

3. *How do you pick a peer mentor?* Choose a colleague whom you trust.

Now that you know what a peer mentor does, you may be wondering why I was so sure I wanted Karen as a peer mentor on this project. We met almost 10 years ago when Karen was a graduate student in our nurse-educator track. Over the years, our mutual trust and respect has grown as Karen has peer mentored me on different presentation projects. Living 10 minutes from one another, we share a love of walking. Fast-paced walks along wooded trails or by the water with Karen's three dogs have become our still-point strategy, a physical way of moving into reflective space so we can plan for presentations. Even though Karen was new to the topic of joy-stealing, I knew that she could make this presentation relevant to this audience of school nurses, because she is a school nurse.

Who are the Karen's in your life? Who are the colleague–friends who listen well, who bring a beginner's mind to topics, whether they're experts or not, and whom you trust. Write the names of one or more individuals who meet these three criteria in Jot Box 32-1.

Jot Box 32-1

Names of Your Potential Peer Mentors

1. _____

2. _____

3. _____

It's fine if you don't have a special someone in mind just yet. While Karen was the obvious choice in this case, it can take me weeks of wracking my brain only to discover the perfect candidate hiding in plain sight. Now that you're on the lookout for a peer mentor, you may begin to see your colleague–friends in a different light. It's a good idea to keep the names of potential peer mentors in your *Dare to Share* notebook. That way, whenever you get a new gig, you can refer to your ever expanding list and streamline the search process.

Every presentation project has both technical and relational aspects. As a presenter, you must learn to attend to each and balance both. Depending on the nature of each step, the remaining chapters in this section address either a technical strategy or skill or a relational support-circle issue.

TIP

A peer mentor, well chosen, is the greatest gift a presenter can ask for.

References

1. Costa, A. L., & Garmston, R. (1992). Cognitive coaching for peer reflection. *Journal of Supervision and Curricular Development, 5*(20), 15–19.
2. Heinrich, K. T., & Scherr, M. (1994, July–August). Peer mentoring for reflective teaching. *Nurse Educator, 19*(4), 36–41.

How to Decide Whether to Go Solo or Co-Present

33

O you who love clear edges more than anything . . . watch the edges that blur.

Adrienne Rich

Around about the time you're deciding on a peer mentor, you'll need to figure out whether you want to go solo or co-present. Sometimes the answer is obvious. If you're sharing your own work, then yours will be a solo presentation. When things aren't so clear-cut, complete the questionnaire in Information Box 33-1.

Let's discuss each question separately. With regard to the first question, if you can complete a presentation without assistance, a decision to co-present is motivated by factors other than need. For example, when you're new to presenting or presenting on a new topic, enlisting someone with name recognition or political connections may be a legitimate reason to consider a co-presenting collaboration.

With regard to the second question, if you work better by yourself going solo takes less time and keeps you in control of the content and quality of the final product. If you enjoy working with others, asking a colleague(s) to co-present may be a good idea. The upside is that you get to split the to-do list. As has been said, the downside is the ratio of prepa-

---

Information Box 33-1

Questionnaire to Determine Solo or Collaborative Presentation

1. What type of assistance do I need from a colleague on this presentation project?
   a. None
   b. Provide specialized knowledge or expertise
   c. Assist with the design
   d. Support during the presenting process
   e. Help with presenting
   f. Offer a professional affiliation or political connection

2. How do I work best?
   a. By myself
   b. With someone else
   c. Not sure

3. What can the colleague I have in mind contribute?
   a. Nothing
   b. Provide specialized knowledge or expertise
   c. Assist with the design
   d. Support during the presenting process
   e. Help with presenting
   f. Offer a professional affiliation or political connection
   g. Give me the opportunity to serve as a mentor

---

ration time to the number of presenters. Calculate preparation time increases in multiples of the number of presenters involved in the project: two presenters take twice as long, three presenters take three times as long, and so on.

When you have a particular person in mind, as I did with Karen, then answering the third question can make the decision for you. When I first spoke with Karen about peer mentoring my presentation, I had a feeling that I might ask her to get involved in the actual presentation. Had I completed this questionnaire at the time, my answers would have been as shown in the box that follows on page 120.

Questionnaire to Determine Solo or Collaborative Presentation

1. What type of assisstance do I need on this presentation project?
   a. Nothing
   ✔ b. Provide specialized knowledge or expertise—*specifically, school nursing*
   ✔ c. Assist with the design—*to tailor content to a school nursing audience*
   d. Support during the presenting process
   e. Help with presenting
   f. Offer a professional affiliation or political connection
2. How do I work best?
   a. By myself
   ✔ b. With someone else
   c. Not sure
3. What can this particular individual—*Karen*—contribute to this presentation?
   a. Nothing
   ✔ b. Provide specialized knowledge or expertise—*Karen is a school nurse.*
   ✔ c. Assist with the design
   ✔ d. Support during the presenting process
   ✔ e. Help with presenting
   ✔ f. Offer a professional affiliation or political connection— *Karen is a member of the group to whom I am presenting.*
   g. Give me the opportunity to serve as a mentor.

Karen's expertise as a school nurse (*specialized knowledge*) and her membership in the group to whom I was presenting (*professional affiliation*) made her the perfect co-presenter. Or did it? You'll find out in the next chapter.

TIP

Clarify your preference for going solo or co-presenting early in the planning process.

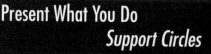
How to Negotiate Mindful Presenting Relationships

34

Go slow. Relationships aren't marathons, they're strolls.

Grandmother to Granddaughter

During our peer mentoring preconference, I asked Karen if she would share a story with the audience about a school nurse in a joy-stealing situation. This made Karen's contribution more than that of a peer mentor and less than that of a co-presenter. Thankfully, there's a way to thank colleagues for assists such as storytelling. It's called an *acknowledgment*. Acknowledgments are in order when someone serves as a technical assistant, a project coordinator, a resource allocator (administrators often fall into this category), a data collector, a data analyzer, an editorial reviewer, or a peer mentor.[1]

With three options—go solo, acknowledge, or co-present—an invitation to consider collaborating on a presentation can be an exploratory negotiation rather than a fait accompli. What if every time you asked a colleague to consider a collaboration you scheduled a meeting to discuss the following three questions?

1. What do I want from my involvement in this presentation project?
2. What can I contribute to this presentation project?
3. What's worked well about presenting or co-presenting in my past?

121

To show you how such a dialogue might go, this is what Karen and I discovered in the course of our exploratory dialogue.

> 1. *What do I want from my involvement in this presentation project?* I wanted the experience of presenting to this group because I have a special place in my heart for school nurses and I welcomed the opportunity to add this group's stories to my collection of joy-stealing stories. Karen wanted to help me out, enjoy the intellectual stimulation we've experienced in our past collaborations, and make a contribution to her school-nurse colleagues.
>
> 2. *What can I contribute to this presentation project?* I contribute my expertise as a presenter and the findings from my research exploring joy-stealing. Karen contributes her experience as a school nurse along with her experience as both a presenter and a peer mentor.
>
> 3. *What's worked well about presenting or co-presenting in my past?* Karen and I are about as different as two people can be, and our differences make us a good team. Karen questions my assumptions, keeps me mindful about what an audience really wants to learn, and contributes creative suggestions for the actual presentation that make it sparkle. We've both been so enriched by our peer-mentoring collaborations that we want to do it again.

Beyond serving as my peer mentor, we agreed that Karen would be acknowledged for telling a story about a school nurse's experience with joy-stealing. After clarifying our roles, we moved into setting a timeline that kept our project on task.

Discussing these questions before committing to a working relationship leaves colleagues free to go solo, to acknowledge contributions, or to co-present. Such dialogues lead to decision making based on mutual respect, compatible working styles, and the substance of contributions to the project. Easterners call such relationships *mindful*; Westerners call them *conscious*. Whether you call them mindful or conscious, the care and maintenance of support circles involves negotiating collaborative relationships that stay collegial throughout the presenting project.

Should you decide to co-present, the next step is negotiating an agreement that includes a contract and a covenant.[1] *Contracts* are agreements that deal with the details of the project, such as the following:

- The order of names of co-presenters
- A list of who is responsible for what
- A Timeline Worksheet with delineated tasks and time frames

Covenants are agreements that describe how co-presenters interact. They can include the following:

- A way to handle disagreements and misunderstandings when they arise
- A pact to renegotiate agreements, as needed

To give your collaboration the best chance of working smoothly, put your contract and covenant in writing and circulate copies to all co-presenters. Although this may strike you as cold and legalistic, clarifying agreements upfront is part of cultivating mindful relationships. Should questions arise, your agreement can serve as a clarification or a jumping off point for renegotiation. It works best to consider such agreements as works in progress (see Chapter 88 for an example of an actual contract/covenant).

With three options on the table, you'll be able to negotiate and renegotiate agreements that reflect and honor colleagues' contributions to presentation projects. Now that we've talked about what you're going to present and who to involve in your presentation, it's time to talk about how to present in a way that turns audiences into participants.

TIP

Negotiate a contract and covenant to keep your working relationship productive and vibrant during presentation projects.

Reference

1. Heinrich, K. T., Pardue, K. T., Davison-Price, M., Murphy, J. I., Neese, R., Walker, P., et al. (2005, January/February). How can I help you? How can you help me?: Transforming nursing education through partnerships. *Nursing Education Perspectives, 26*(1), 34–41.

How to Design Presentations That Show and Tell

35

Tell me and I'll forget. Show me and I may not remember. Involve me and I'll understand.

Native American saying

Not long ago, a colleague said that she doesn't see much difference between paper presentations and workshops at nursing conferences. She's so right. Good presenters, like good creative writers, show and then tell. Although there should be a huge difference between delivering a paper and facilitating a workshop, when presenters are tall on tell and short on show, presentations all look alike. To see what a show-and-tell presentation looks like, read Gina's outline for her 20-minute presentation on stress for her 14 undergraduate classmates.

Gina's soda-can experiment was a brilliant maneuver. After getting us to stress, she asked what we experienced as we opened our soda cans. In the process, *we* ended up listing all the symptoms of stress identified in the literature. In choosing a coping strategy for the week, we applied what we had learned about stress to our own lives.

Gina based her show-and-tell presentation on Kolb's experiential learning cycle.[1] When David Kolb, a university professor, began consulting, he found that business people would become fidgety whenever he started presentations with his usual facts and figures. Because he

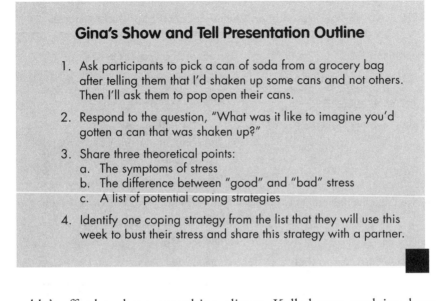

Gina's Show and Tell Presentation Outline

1. Ask participants to pick a can of soda from a grocery bag after telling them that I'd shaken up some cans and not others. Then I'll ask them to pop open their cans.

2. Respond to the question, "What was it like to imagine you'd gotten a can that was shaken up?"

3. Share three theoretical points:
   a. The symptoms of stress
   b. The difference between "good" and "bad" stress
   c. A list of potential coping strategies

4. Identify one coping strategy from the list that they will use this week to bust their stress and share this strategy with a partner.

couldn't afford to bore consulting clients, Kolb began studying how adults learn. In addition to learning differently, he found that adults learn from life experiences that violate their expectations and introduce them to a new worldview. Kolb identified four learning styles and developed a learning cycle to address each style, beginning with participants engaging in a "concrete experience" (CE); reflecting on that experience during "reflective observation" (RO); learning the theory related to the problem during "abstract conceptualization" (AC); and applying what they've learned to their lives during active experimentation (AE).

Table 35-1 shows how the four phases in Gina's presentation fit with Kolb's experiential learning model stages.

Let's define Kolb's terms and link them to the learning activities in Gina's presentation:

- **Concrete Experience (CE):** Learners engage in a hands-on activity related to the topic. Notice how Gina's CE actively engages participants in a stressful exercise when they don't know whether their can of soda was shaken.
- **Reflective Observation (RO):** Learners reflect on what it was like to participate in the concrete experience. In Gina's presentation,

TABLE 35-1   Gina's Presentation Outline Incorporating Kolb's Stages

Presentation Title	"Stress-Less Coping Strategies"
Concrete Experience (CE)	Soda can experiment
Reflective Observation (RO)	What was that like for you?
Abstract Conceptualization (AC)	Three important points: • The symptoms of stress • "Good" versus "bad" stress • Potential coping strategies
Active Experimentation (AE)	Write an affirmation: This week, I commit to using _____ coping strategy.
Reflective Observation (RO)	What was that like for you?

during the RO, participants consider what it was like to feel the stress of not knowing.

- **Abstract Conceptualization (AC):** Only those theoretical points specific to the slant are introduced during the AC. In Gina's presentation, participants are introduced to three key points related to stress-less coping strategies.
- **Active Experimentation (AE):** Learners apply what they've learned to their own situations. Gina's AE activity allows participants to commit to using a specific coping strategy learned during the AC.
- **Reflective Observation (RO):** Because participants like to reflect on AEs, I took the advice of an educator who adds an RO after the AE. From now on, you'll see an RO in all Kolb's Model sequences *both* after the CE *and* after the AE.

I hope that David Kolb is flattered to learn that my students have turned his name into a verb. To *Kolb* a presentation is to make it a show-and-tell experience. Using Gina's outline as a guide, it's time for you to turn your eye-glittering idea into a show-and-tell presentation.

Your Kolb-It Worksheet

Idea: Stress

Snappy Title: Stress-Less Coping Strategies

CE: Soda can experiment.

RO: What was it like to imagine you'd gotten a soda can that was shaken up?

AC:

- The symptoms of stress
- The difference between "good" and "bad" stress
- Coping strategies

AE: Free-write one coping strategy from the ones listed that you will use this week to bust your stress and share this strategy with a partner.

RO: What was it like to identify and share your coping strategy?

Your Kolb-It

Idea: _____

Snappy Title: _____

CE (Design an exercise that involves learners in their own learning.):

_____

_____

(continues)

Your Kolb-It Worksheet (continued)

RO (Ask learners to reflect on the concrete experience.): What was

that like for you?

AC (Highlight salient theoretical points.):

_____

_____

_____

_____

AE (Allow learners to apply learning to their lives.):

_____

RO (What was that like for you?):

_____

What was it like to *Kolb* your presentation? Reading about the technique and then using it to frame your focused idea for a presentation are two different things. Did it hurt your head and cramp your style? If this is your first time Kolb-ing and you got frustrated, you're right where you should be. Be patient with yourself. It's always hard to try something different.

If you're feeling frustrated, can you imagine how a nursing audience used to tell-and-show presentations feels after a show-and-tell presentation? Nurses may find an interactive learning experience enjoyable in the moment, but once it's over they ask themselves what they've learned. When they assess a show-and-tell presentation using tell-and-show criteria, the show-and-tell always comes up short. That's why it is important to tell your audience upfront that you're shifting the rules. Make it safe and intriguing by inviting them to "try something new."[2] I say something like, "If it's one thing I know about adult learners, it's that we don't like being lectured to. We much prefer to share our rich life experiences. So today, I'm not going to talk at you, we're going to learn from one another." When approached in this manner, most nursing audiences are game. As you and your audiences experience the magic unleashed whenever they become participants, you will all begin to appreciate the value of interactive learning, and show-and-tell presentations may become your signature.

TIP
Flip It! Design presentations that show first and then tell.

References

1. Kolb, D. (1984). *Experiential learning: Experience as the source of learning and development.* Englewood Cliffs, NJ: Prentice Hall.
2. Ironside, P. M. (2003). Trying something new: Implementing and evaluative narrative pedagogy using a multi-method approach. *Nursing Education Perspectives, 24*, 122–128.

How to Kolb
Longer Presentations

36

*Creativity can be defined as
letting go of certainties.*

Gail Sheehy

Gina's presentation in the last chapter was 20 minutes long. What do you do when a presentation needs to last longer than 20 minutes? This chapter shows you how to design longer presentations by "cycling" Kolb's learning cycle. This approach allows you to expand Kolb's model to fit presentations of any time frame while maintaining a show-and-tell format. As you can see below, Karen and I designed a two-cycle show-and-tell design for our 1-hour presentation for the school nurses.

Design for Cycle 1

Title: Joy-Stealing Games: What School Nurses Can Do to Stop the Game-Playing

Cycle 1

    CE: Karen's joy-stealing story
    RO: What was it like to hear Karen's story?
    AC: Four roles: target, joy-stealer, bystander, ally
    AE: What roles did you hear in Karen's story?
    RO: What was it like for you to identify those roles?

The first cycle allowed participants to learn about the four roles played in joy-stealing games by linking them with the characters described in Karen's story.

Design for Cycle 2

Cycle 2

CE: Free-write: Write about a situation with a student, teacher, administrator, or parent(s) that is stealing your joy.
RO: What was it like for you to write your story?
AC:

Strategies:
- Empower targets.
- Increase empathy in perpetrators.
- Encourage bystanders to become allies.

Healing measures:
- Become an ally to yourself.
- Become an ally to students.
- Become an ally to colleagues, to parents, and to administrators.

AE: Share stories.
Affirmation: I commit to becoming an ally to myself in dealing with my joy-stealing situation by . . .
RO: What was it like for you to make this affirmation?

Whereas Karen's story about a school nurse allowed the audience to learn the various roles played in joy-stealing games, the second cycle allowed participants to tell their own stories and to strategize how to deal with joy-stealing situations. The show of the stories combined with the tell of joy-stealing theory enabled participants to apply their learning to their practices. For school nurses, who are doers by nature, it doesn't get any better than that.

In Kolb's terms, you can see how the CE and AE activities in our first cycle prepared participants for the CE and the AE in our second cycle. Part of the fun and challenge of cycling Kolb's model is playing with CE and AE activities to come up with the combinations that best engage participants in their own learning. The following is a list of activities suitable for either CEs or AEs:

- Quiz
- Video/film clip

- Song
- Game
- Role play
- Dialogue question
- Experiment
- Storytelling
- Free-write

The following is a shorthand version that allowed us to mix and match and compare and contrast CE and AE exercises in the first and second cycle.

Cycle 1
CE: Karen's joy-stealing story
AE: Match roles with Karen's characters

Cycle 2
CE: Audience free-writes
AE: Audience share stories

Although this shorthand comparison is useful in the planning stage, the only way to assess the power of a CE–AE combination is to test it in actual presentations until participants' responses lead you to the most effective CE–AE combination.

Now it's your turn to design a longer presentation. Building on the CE–AE learning activities you identified in the last chapter, develop a two-cycle, Kolb's model design for a 1-hour presentation.

Your Two-Cycle Design
Cycle 1
CE: _____
RO: _____
AC: _____
AE: _____
RO: _____
(continues)

Your Two-Cycle Design (continued)

Cycle 2

CE: _____

RO: _____

AC: _____

AE: _____

RO: _____

How was that for you?

Although it can be a bit confusing at first, the cycling concept ensures that a presentation stays interactive regardless of its length. Say you're planning a weekend workshop. The final learning cycle of the first day ends with an AE journal writing assignment for participants to complete as a homework assignment; the next morning begins with an RO about what it was like to complete the journal assignment. Then a new Kolb's cycle starting with a CE initiates the process all over again.

The next chapter offers another way to ensure that all the moving parts in your presentation work together to create a cohesive whole.

TIP

For every 20 minutes of presentation, use a Kolb's cycle to keep presentations show and tell.

How to Ensure that Presentations Are Internally Consistent

37

> *It's not true that life is one damn thing after another. . . . It's the same damn thing over and over again.*
>
> Edna St. Vincent Millay

Although repetition in everyday life may be tedious, the repetition of a slant makes for a presentation that is coherent and cohesive. Such a presentation is said to be *internally consistent*. As you know from the Presentation Worksheet, a slant is introduced in the title. In Kolb's model, slants are experienced in the CE, reflected upon in the RO, theorized about in the AC, applied in the AE to participants' lives, and reflected upon again in the final RO. Notice how in both cycles of our presentation the slant of "joy-stealing" runs from the title and through the CE straight through to the final RO.

Internal Consistency Checklist

Cycle 1

Idea: *Joy-stealing* games
Title: *Joy-Stealing* Games: How School Nurses Can Become Allies for Themselves

> **CE**: Karen's *joy-stealing* story
> **RO**: What was it like to hear Karen's story?
> **AC**: *Four roles in joy-stealing games*: target, joy stealer, bystander, ally
> **AE**: What *joy-stealing* roles did you hear in Karen's story?
> **RO**: What was it like for you to identify roles in *joy-stealing games*?

Cycle 2

> **CE**: Free-write: Write about a situation with a student, teacher, administrator, or parent(s) that is *stealing your joy.*
> **RO**: What was it like to write about your *joy-stealing story*?
> **AC**:
> Strategies that *bust joy-stealing:*
> - Empower targets.
> - Increase empathy in perpetrators.
> - Encourage bystanders to become allies.
>
> Strategies to *recover zest:*
> - Become an ally to yourself.
> - Become an ally to students.
> - Become an ally to colleagues, to parents, and to administrators.
>
> **AE**: Share stories
> Affirmation: I commit to becoming an ally to myself in *dealing with my joy-stealing situation* by . . .
> **RO**: What was that like for you to make this affirmation?

In a presentation that's internally consistent, the slant is the unifying theme that repeats throughout. Now it's your turn to make sure there's a single and consistent theme that runs from your idea to your title and through the stages in your Kolb's model.

Your Internal Consistency Check

Idea: _____

_____

_____

Snappy Title: _____

_____

_____

CE: _____

_____

_____

RO: _____

_____

_____

AC: _____

_____

_____

AE: _____

_____

_____

RO: _____

_____

_____

Once you verify that your presentation design is internally consistent, you're ready to translate your design into a presentation packet that's a valuable take-away for attendees as you will see in Chapter 39. Before designing your packet, however, you'd do well to assess your audience's response.

TIP

An internally consistent Kolb's model presentation is an art form that leaves audiences with a satisfied sense of completion.

How to Assess
Audience Response

38

*Assessment will gradually become an integral
part of every [presenter's] reflective practice.*

Peter T. Ewell[1]

You can turn your audience members into active participants by asking them for their response to your presentation. Audience-participants' responses can be gauged in three ways: through numbers (quantitative), stories (qualitative), or a combination of both. There is no right or wrong way. Choosing an assessment strategy is a matter of presenter preference, and the following describes my own preference.

What do I want to learn from assessment data? I want to know what participants liked and would change about my presentation and why.

Will numbers, stories, or a combination of both tell me what I want to know? Stories will give me the best sense of what I want to know.

To help you decide on an assessment approach that fits you and your style, this chapter offers three possibilities, citing the pros and cons of each. The first is an example of a quantitative approach in which close-ended questions elicit yes-no answers. Arranged along a continuum, called a Likert scale, responses can be translated into the percentage of respondents who strongly agree, agree, disagree, or strongly disagree.

Presenter was knowledgeable.

1	2	3	4
Strongly Agree	Agree	Disagree	Strongly Disagree

Quantitative Assessment Item

Pro: Numerical percentages convey general audience trends.
Con: No rationale provided for individual participant's responses.

The second option is an example of a qualitative approach that asks open-ended questions that elicit respondents' free-writes:

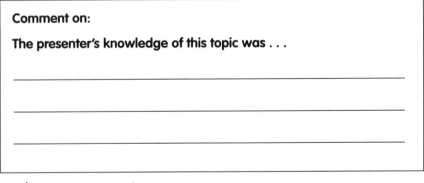

Comment on:

The presenter's knowledge of this topic was . . .

Qualitative Assessment Item

Pro: Participants' respond to specific topics and offer rationales for their responses.
Con: Specific topics may or may not yield information relevant to presenters.

The most informative results can come from assessment surveys that combine quantitative and qualitative approaches. See how the following example includes a closed-ended statement, and a request for comments to explain the numeric rating.

Presenter was knowledgeable.

1	2	3	4

◄──►

Strongly   Agree   Disagree   Strongly
Agree   Disagree

Comments:

_____

_____

_____

Quantitative/Qualitative Combo Assessment Item

Pro: Allows presenters to verify the congruence between numerical scores and narrative comments; for example, if someone circles "4" and writes that the presenter was knowledgeable, the presenter knows they meant to circle "1."

Con: None that I can think of.

Now that you're familiar with the three possibilities, I'll share the qualitative approach that gives me the feedback I need to refine presentations. My one-page evaluation form asks participants to respond to three specific questions adapted from Peggy's Chinn's[2] "check-out" questions: (1) appreciation, (2) critique, and (3) affirmation. The following is the evaluation sheet that's included in all my presentation packets.

Audience Response Assessment Sheet

Check Out/Evaluation

Name of Offering: _____

Date of Offering: _____

Appreciation of this learning experience:

_____

_____

_____

Critique to make this presentation better:

_____

_____

_____

Affirmation: Based on what I've learned, my next step is . . .

_____

_____

_____

Now that you know the pros and cons of each assessment approach, you're ready to answer these two questions for yourself (Jot Box 38-1).

Jot Box 38-1

What do I want to learn from assessment data?

_____

_____

Will numbers, stories, or a combination of both tell me what I want to know?

_____

_____

Consider your assessment approach as much of a personal signature as your presenting style. Start by collecting assessment forms from every class and conference session you attend. Then try them out. Give audiences 5 minutes at the end of every presentation to complete assessments to see which one, or which combination, you prefer. Once you find your favorite format, you'll have all you need to refine each presentation for next time.

TIP

Evaluation is a considerate act that raises your audience awareness quotient.

References

1. Ewell, P.T. (2002). An emerging scholarship: A brief history of assessment. In T.W. Banta & Associates, *Building a scholarship of assessment.* San Francisco: Jossey-Bass.
2. Chinn, P. (2004). *Peace and power: Creative leadership for building community* (6th ed.). Sudbury, MA: Jones and Bartlett.

How to Perk Up Presentation Packets

39

*Creativity requires both imagination
and precision . . .*

Julia Cameron

Let me tell you the never-ending story of my packet from Suzanne Hall Johnson's 1979 publishing workshop. I filed it away and never looked at it again until 1984 when I was writing my first manuscript. In 1994, I pulled it out again to help me design a publication workshop. In 2005, it was listed as a reference in our article on preparing students to write for publication.[1] Today, it sits next to me as I write *Dare to Share*, almost 30 years after Suzanne first handed it to me.

A well-designed packet is a "take away" that participants save. Maybe that's why I always give participants a presentation packet, whether it's a one-page worksheet or a 25-page document complete with references. This chapter shares the packet for our presentation to the school nurse group to use as a guide in preparing your own packet. Skim the items contained on the Presentation Packet Checklist.

143

Presentation Packet Checklist

___ **1. Title page**
 ___ a. Presentation title
 ___ b. Presenter's name, credentials, and affiliation
 ___ c. Date of presentation
 ___ d. Venue/location of presentation
 ___ e. Acknowledgements/appreciations
 ___ f. Presenter's contact information (phone, e-mail address, Web site)

___ **2. Essential information about the learning experience**
 ___ a. Description of the learning experience
 ___ b. Learning objective(s)
 ___ c. Presenter's bio
 ___ d. Session schedule

___ **3. Worksheet(s)**

___ **4. Evaluation form and checkout**

___ **5. Reference list**

___ **6. PowerPoint slides**

___ **7. Participant's contact information (Optional)**

As you read through my presentation packet, see which items on this checklist are included in my packet.

Joy-Stealing Games:
What School Nurses Can Do to Stop the Game-Playing

Kathleen T. Heinrich, RN, PhD
Principal, K T H Consulting

Association of School Nurses Of Connecticut
Fall Dinner Meeting

Thursday, October 26, 2006

Country House Restaurant
East Haven, CT

Acknowledgments

To Karen Owen RN, MSN for her peer mentoring, story telling, and guidance in fitting our presentation to our audience.

To Marji Lipshez-Shapiro for creating the "Names Can Really Hurt" program.

Joy-Stealing Games:
What School Nurses Can Do to Stop the Game-Playing

Kathleen T. Heinrich, RN, PhD

Session Description: Designed to stimulate spirited dialogue, this interactive session engages participants in sharing stories about students, teachers, administrators and parent(s) joy-stealers and strategizing new ways of responding that foster zestful academic environments.

Objective: After this workshop, participants will initiate a dialogue about how school nurses can foster zestful school environments with zero-tolerance for joy-stealing games.

Presenter Bio: Kathleen T. Heinrich, PhD is an award winning educator, prolific author, and popular speaker. The principal of **K T H Consulting**, she consults with nursing groups on fostering zestful workplaces. In addition to consulting, Kathleen is writing a book called *A Nurse's Guide for Presenting and Publishing: Dare to Share* for Jones and Bartlett Publishers.

Session Schedule:

7:00–7:05	Greetings and Set the Stage
7:05–7:15	Karen's Story & Four Roles Played
	Target
	Joy-Stealer
	Bystander
	Ally
7:15–7:25	Free-writes/Roles Played
7:25–7:50	Stop the Joy-Stealing and Restore the Zest Strategies
7:50–8:00	Checkout & Affirmations

Free-write:

Write about a situation with a student, teacher, administrator, or parent(s) that is stealing your joy . . .

_____

_____

_____

_____

_____

_____

Roles Played:

Target: _____

Joy-Stealer: _____

Bystander: _____

Ally: _____

**Please tear off and submit to Kathy
so your story can help stop the joy-stealing.**

Definitions:

Civility: ". . . implies respect for others, a willingness to hear each other's views, and the exercise of restraint in criticizing the views and actions of others" (Higher Education Research Institute, 1996).

Horizontal violence: "Horizontal violence is harmful behavior, via attitudes, actions, words, and other behaviors that is directed towards us by another colleague. Horizontal violence controls, humiliates, denigrates or injures the dignity of another. Horizontal violence indicates a lack of mutual respect and value for the worth of the individual and denies another's fundamental human rights" (Blanton, Lybecker, & Spring, 1998, Definition section, ¶2).

Joy-stealing: Experiences with students, teachers, administrators and parents that rob nurses ". . . of their zest, clarity, productivity, feelings of worth, and desire for more connection" (Heinrich, 2006).

"Names Can Really Hurt" High School Assembly Program (Shapiro, 2006):

Goals. To:
- Empower targets
- Teach empathy to joy-stealers
- Challenge bystanders to become allies

Healing Strategy. Become ally to:
- Yourself
- Students
- Teachers
- Administrators
- Parents

References

Blanton, B. A., Lybecker, C., & Spring, N. M. (1998, July). *A horizontal violence position statement.* Retrieved May 19, 2006, from http://members.shaw.ca/raestonehouse/horizontal_violence_position_s.htm

Heinrich, K. T. (2006, Third Quarter). Joy-stealing: How some nurse educators resist these faculty games. *Reflections on Nursing Leadership.* Available at: http://www.nursingsociety.org

Heinrich, K. T. (2006, Second Quarter). Joy-stealing games. *Reflections on Nursing Leadership.* Available at: http://www.nursingsociety.org

Higher Education Research Institute, UCLA (1996). A Social Change Model for Leadership Development, Version III, Regents of the University of California.

Hirshey, G. (2007, January 28). Pushing back at bullying. Connecticut and the Region. *The New York Times, 14,* 1, 8.

Shapiro, M. (2006, September). *Names can really hurt.* Anti-Defamation League. Available at: http://www.adl.org

Let me be the change I want to see free write:

Affirmation: I commit to becoming an ally to myself in dealing with my joy-stealing situation by . . .

Joy-Stealing Games:
What School Nurses Can Do to Stop the Game-Playing

Checkout/Final Evaluation

Appreciation of this Program:

_____

_____

_____

_____

_____

Critique to improve this program:

_____

_____

_____

_____

_____

Affirmation: I commit to becoming an ally to myself in dealing with my joy-stealing situation by . . .

Tear off and submit to Kathy.

Joy-Stealing Games:
What School Nurses Can Do to Stop the Game-Playing

Participant List

Name	Telephone	Email Address

As you can see from the items checked off below, most of the items on the checklist appear in my packet.

Presentation Packet Checklist

✓ 1. **Title page**
    ✓ a. Presentation title
    ✓ b. Presenter's name, credentials, and affiliation
    ✓ c. Date of presentation
    ✓ d. Venue/location of presentation
    ✓ e. Acknowledgments/appreciations
    ✓ f. Presenter's contact information (phone, e-mail address, Web site URL)

✓ 2. **Essential information about the learning experience**
    ✓ a. Description of learning experience
    ✓ b. Learning objective(s): In specific, measurable, behavioral terms
    ✓ c. Presenter's Bio: Background information related to presentation
    ✓ d. Schedule overview: Topics and time frames

✓ 3. **Body of packet**
    a. Homework assignment
    ✓ b. Worksheet(s)
    ✓ c. Reference list (if applicable)
    d. PowerPoint slides (if applicable)
    e. Homework assignment to complete for next time
    ✓ f. Evaluation form and checkout
    ✓ g. Participant's contact information (Optional)

Now it's your turn. Enjoy creating your own presentation packet using this checklist as a guide. In Chapter 40, I've asked Melissa Dayton, my personal PowerPoint maven, who also happens to be my neighbor, friend, and walking buddy, to share the secrets she's learned about designing PowerPoint presentations in her years as an educator of adults.

■
TIP
Create presentation packets with imagination and precision.

References

1. Heinrich, K. T., Pardue, K. T., Davison-Price, M., Murphy, J. I., Neese, R., Walker, R., et al. (2005, January/February). How can I help you? How can you help me?: Transforming nursing education through partnerships. *Nursing Education Perspectives, 26*(1), 34–41.

How to Power Up
Your Use of PowerPoint

40

Melissa Dayton, MM, MA

*PowerPoint has all sorts of power built into it,
but it turns out the hardest thing is to keep it
simple, and I think people connect with simple.*

Lawrence Lessig

PowerPoint displays can draw accolades or groans, smiles or yawns, exhilaration or dread, on the part of presenters and audience members alike. Before you step into your presenter shoes, think back to a presentation you attended that featured a PowerPoint display to answer the questions in Jot Box 40-1.

If your experience was a positive one, that's great! If, however, you don't remember much about it or the presentation left you cold, don't blame PowerPoint! It's the presenter who designed a display that was unfocused, poorly organized, or just plain dull.

Much more than a death by drone compounded by bullet points, PowerPoint when used well can enhance your message and make it accessible to all members of your audience. PowerPoint displays can be a compelling facet of presentations that keep your audience's attention engaged and focused on you and your message. Before we get underway, let's talk about what you will and won't learn from reading this chapter.

You *won't* learn how to use PowerPoint. For those of you who are new to PowerPoint, there are many ways to learn how to use the program. The

---

Jot Box 40-1

1. **What do you remember about the presentation?**

   _____

   _____

2. **What did you like about it?**

   _____

   _____

3. **What didn't you like about it?**

   _____

   _____

---

hands-on tutorial included with PowerPoint can walk you through the basics. Books about PowerPoint are readily available online and at bookstores. And, if you are the do-it-yourself type, simply open a blank PowerPoint file and dive in!

You *will* learn how PowerPoint can be used to bolster, clarify, and enliven a presentation by seeing how it enriches Kathy's presentation on joy-stealing. In this text, we use the term *PowerPoint* to refer to any type of slide-based presentation software (e.g., Apple's Keynote presentation software). Instead of referring to PowerPoint *presentations,* we'll talk about PowerPoint *displays* to emphasize that PowerPoint is but one element in your overall presentation.

To PowerPoint or Not to PowerPoint: That Is the Question

Now that you've completed your Presentation Worksheet and Kolbed your presentation, you're ready to consider the PowerPoint decision. To make this decision, add your responses to the five questions in the Item Completion Box, using Kathy's presentation on joy-stealing as a guide.

Item Completion Box

1. **What's the slant/title of your presentation? ?**

   Kathy's: <u>Joy Stealing: What School Nurses Can Do to Stop</u>

   <u>the Mean Games</u>

   Yours: _____

2. **What's the purpose of your presentation?**

   Kathy's: <u>Educate and move to action</u>

   Yours: _____

3. **What's the desired audience response?**

   Kathy's: <u>Foster zestful school environments with zero-</u>

   <u>tolerance for such games.</u>

   Yours: _____

4. **What's the venue?**

   Kathy's: <u>A restaurant dining room</u>

   Yours: _____

5. **What's the format for your presentation?**

   Kathy's: <u>*Interactive format, including storytelling, audience*</u>

   <u>*response, the introduction of new concepts and strategies, a*</u>

   <u>*free-write activity, and a personal statement of affirmation.*</u>

   Yours: _____

After reviewing these five items, Kathy concludes that that the only impediment to using PowerPoint is the venue, which is a restaurant dining area. She'll have to check with the conference convener about whether PowerPoint is even an option. Even though this presentation is far from a traditional lecture, Kathy could use PowerPoint to visually enhance and facilitate learning by employing some of the following elements:

- An engaging, intriguing, or provocative quote to set the tone for the presentation and start the audience thinking about the topic
- A brief agenda or summary of purpose so participants know what to expect of the workshop
- An attractive photo or other image that provides a visual backdrop to Karen's story
- A bulleted slide(s) that summarize the joy-stealing concepts and strategies to highlight key points in Kathy's spoken presentation and provide a "hook" for visual learners
- An instructional prompt for the free-write activity that participants can refer to as they work

Revisit your own Presentation Worksheet. Perhaps you are introducing colleagues to new equipment or a new skill set, providing a status report at a meeting, presenting a paper at a conference, or exhibiting a poster at a health fair. Can PowerPoint help you format your presentation to get your desired audience response? Complete the five-question quiz on the following page using Kathy's responses as a guide.

Once you've finished the quiz, tally the number of "yes" responses. If, like Kathy, you answered two or more of these questions with a yes, you're ready to develop a PowerPoint outline.

Develop a PowerPoint Outline

A general PowerPoint outline helps to keep your presentation focus and purpose in mind, as well as curb the temptation to create a new slide for every good idea you have. Kathy's PowerPoint outline is displayed in Information Box 40-1.

Kathy's outline is relatively brief because most of the learning in her interactive presentation will take place "off screen." The following list

To PowerPoint or Not Quiz

1. **Can PowerPoint clarify and enhance the overall structure of your presentation?**

   Kathy: Yes

   You: _____

2. **Can PowerPoint visually highlight or reinforce the essential points you want the audience to take away?**

   Kathy: Yes

   You: _____

3. **Can a PowerPoint treatment facilitate learning at various stages in Kolb's model?**

   Kathy: Yes, particularly in the theory portion (AC) of
   the presentation.

   You: _____

4. **Can PowerPoint provide visual "bursts" that effectively (and affectively) engage, intrigue, provoke, or amuse your audience?**

   Kathy: Yes

   You: _____

5. **Can PowerPoint help you to address your audience's diverse learning styles?**

   Kathy: Yes

   You: _____

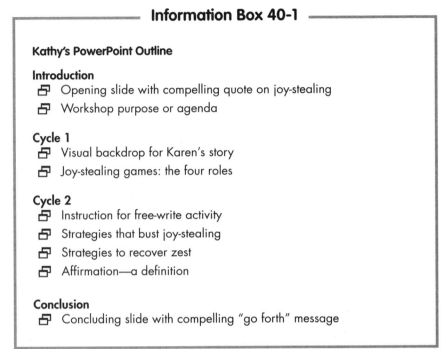

Information Box 40-1

Kathy's PowerPoint Outline

Introduction
- Opening slide with compelling quote on joy-stealing
- Workshop purpose or agenda

Cycle 1
- Visual backdrop for Karen's story
- Joy-stealing games: the four roles

Cycle 2
- Instruction for free-write activity
- Strategies that bust joy-stealing
- Strategies to recover zest
- Affirmation—a definition

Conclusion
- Concluding slide with compelling "go forth" message

suggests a variety of ways to create an outline. Use the way that you find to be quickest and easiest:

- Write directly in PowerPoint using the Outline view.
- Represent your outline in a "skeleton" series of slides that contains titles only.
- Type your outline on a word processor.
- Use pen and paper.
- Use small notecards to jot down ideas that can be arranged in outline form.
- Return to your own Presentation Worksheet to create your own PowerPoint outline.

The process of creating an outline helps to clarify which points can be conveyed in PowerPoint and which can be delivered using other means, such as a presentation packet. Resist the temptation to get too detailed too soon as you develop your own PowerPoint outline in Jot Box 40-2.

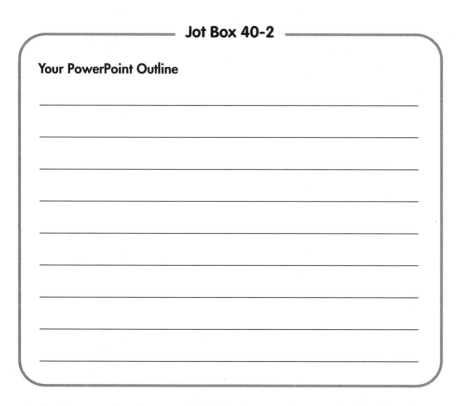

Jot Box 40-2

Your PowerPoint Outline

Flesh-out Your Outline with Content

Once your outline is complete, you're ready to flesh it out with content to include in the PowerPoint display. As you can see from Kathy's outline in Table 40-1, PowerPoint can lend structure to presentations by providing a visual framework or skeleton.

Audience members like to know what to expect and "where they are" during a presentation, much like following the acts or movements of a live performance. Structuring slides orient audience participants throughout the presentation by:

- Introducing you and your presentation
- Outlining your agenda and session objectives
- Announcing the start of a new section or signifying a change in activity
- Summarizing the main points of a section
- Concluding your presentation with a parting thought or call to action

---

TABLE 40-1 Kathy's PowerPoint Slide Display Outline

Basic Outline	**PowerPoint Slide Display**
Introduction	
Opening slide with compelling quote on joy-stealing	A quote that grabs audience attention and sets the scene for what is to come. "You must learn to tolerate that which you allow."
Workshop purpose or agenda	Basic premise of workshop and what participants will take from it.
Cycle 1	
Visual backdrop for Karen's story	Could be picture of playground, Karen, nurses (decide whether to include).
Joy-stealing games: the four roles	Bulleted slides, one slide per role with clarifying info *or* one slide showing all four roles.
Cycle 2	
Instruction for free-write activity	Simple, succinct prompt.
Strategies that bust joy-stealing	One slide per strategy, with examples of each strategy.
Strategies to recover zest	One slide per strategy, with examples of each strategy.
Affirmation—a definition	Common definition. Perhaps display *after* participants have offered their definitions.
Conclusion	
Concluding slide with compelling "go forth" message	Either an affirmative quote to bracket the opening quote or a message of encouragement to "go for the zest."

The PowerPoint content in the joy-stealing presentation example is very simple. Now it's your turn (use Jot Box 40-3). Your expanded outline will reflect *your* presentation and how you have decided to communicate your message.

Jot Box 40-3

Your PowerPoint Slide Display Outline

_____

_____

_____

_____

_____

_____

_____

_____

_____

PowerPoint also provides the flexibility for you to represent and accentuate content in a variety of ways:

- Bullet points communicate key points in a straightforward, easy-to-read manner.
- Quotations express an illustrative or provocative point of view.
- Colorful charts and graphs convey survey results, trends, and other types of data.
- Visual elements such as clip art, photos, and drawings can illustrate or accent a concept or key point.
- Live Web links enable you to display Web sites on the screen and then return to your PowerPoint display.
- Audio and video clips add a multimedia dimension.
- Animation features allow you to control how and when items appear on a slide and create timed slideshows.

Not surprisingly, it's easy to get caught up in this wealth of visual possibilities.

There is no single formula for using PowerPoint. By keeping your presentation focus, purpose, desired audience response, and venue in mind, you're more likely to create a PowerPoint display that supports and propels your presentation.

Design Tips

Audience awareness is key to making your PowerPoint display easy and enjoyable to view. Consider the following when designing your slides:

- Match the background design for your slides to the composition of your audience and your topic. A PowerPoint display featuring school or sports imagery that's age appropriate for a presentation to fifth graders on personal hygiene might be too basic or juvenile for a presentation to a group of healthcare professionals.
- Choose a font scheme and stay consistent. PowerPoint automatically creates a text hierarchy: titles are largest, followed by bullet points, then subpoints. You might, for example, use a 36-point font for headings, 28-point for main bullet points, 24-point for subpoints, and 20-point for citations. The inconsistent or arbitrary use of fonts can distract the visually inclined and confuse those who rely on consistent structure to follow your presentation.
- Keep words on slides to a minimum. When there are too many words on a slide, the slide is difficult to read and won't reproduce well as a handout. Either make your point using multiple slides or provide information as a full-sized handout in your presentation packet.
- Consider the needs of viewers with visual, learning, or other disabilities by following ADA (Americans with Disabilities Act) accessibility guidelines. General principles include:
  - Use a clear, easy-to-read font.
  - Use consistent formatting.
  - Use good color contrast between text and background.
  - Minimize the use of extraneous or "busy" detail.
- Use humor to create an informal atmosphere. This can disarm the biases and preconceptions that participants sometimes bring to presentations. Pictures, cartoons or text can inject a visual burst of surprise into your presentation.

- Experiment with incorporating live web links, audio and video clips, and PowerPoint animation features to support your presentation.
- Provide PowerPoint handouts for participants. PowerPoint handouts that block out the presentation clearly and that provide room for audiences to take notes become a reference document for follow-up, future use, and further exploration.

Edit, Rehearse, and Revise

As you scan your expanded outline, you may decide that some slides are unnecessary, whereas others seem to be missing. One of the beauties of PowerPoint is that editing is easy. You can rearrange slides, delete unwanted slides and insert new ones, and move text and graphic elements among slides. Presenters tend to err on the side of too many slides. Thinking of PowerPoint as a vehicle for—not the driver of—your presentation may help you to pare down your slideshow.

Once your display is as you want it, take the time to rehearse your presentation. This is important. Practicing your presentation, preferably with another person—colleague–friend, peer mentor, co-presenter or supportive family member—allows you to refine your timing, smooth rough spots, get comfortable with PowerPoint technology, and make transitions seamless as you move between presentation, PowerPoint slides, and presentation packet.

When it's not possible to rehearse with someone else, review your PowerPoint display in Slide Show mode to see how your presentation flows and appears to the audience. A slide that makes sense on the small screen may suddenly appear awkward, unclear, or out of context on the "large screen." Rehearsal is particularly important when you're co-presenting, because the success of your presentation depends on your ability to stay coordinated, on time, and on topic.

Tips for Taking Your PowerPoint Display on the Road

To ensure that your presentation runs smoothly, be sure to:

- Bring a backup copy of your file on a flash drive or CD.
- Check compatibility. Although computer systems are generally compatible, it is possible that another computer,

whether PC or Macintosh, will not recognize your Power-Point document.

- Get to the presentation venue early. Most technology glitches can be sorted out when you allow ample time to set up and summon technical help, if necessary.
- Stay calm! If something goes wrong while you are presenting, refer to your handouts, switch gears, and keep the focus on the presentation. By remaining (or at least appearing) unruffled, you will help the audience shift gears with you.

Conclusion

Whether you're novice or expert at creating PowerPoint displays, keep a beginner's mind. After all the PowerPoint displays I've designed, I still see new applications of PowerPoint that stir me to expand my repertoire. The more you practice and present, the more refined your PowerPoint sense will become as you discover new ways to use this powerful tool to communicate your ideas and inspire audiences. Taking what you've learned in Chapters 39 and 40, you're now ready to combine packets and PowerPoint slide displays to enhance participants' learning during and following your presentations. Now it's time to consider adding peer mentors to your support circle by discussing the steps involved in developing peer-mentoring relationships with colleague–friends.

TIP
Use PowerPoint slide displays to enhance the visual appeal and learning potential of your presentations.

How to Prepare *Who* Questions for Pre-Sessions with Peer Mentors

41

Desire, ask, believe, receive.

Stella Terrill Mann

You've chosen your peer mentor and set aside a mutually convenient hour and 15 minutes for a pre-presentation session. What now? I can't count the number of times that I've said to my peer mentor, "I'm in great shape with this presentation. Our pre-session should take about a half hour." Only to spend an hour together discussing the presentation and a couple of hours afterwards incorporating changes to what I thought was a done deal. Consider this a loving warning. The very act of having an interested listener whose only job is to help you sift through who you are as a presenter, what you want to present, and how you want to present is a reflective practice-in-relationship.[1,2] A well-chosen peer mentor helps you to step outside yourself to see your presentation through the eyes of a sympathetic other who is somewhere between a stand-in for your audience and a wise observer.

Between your desire for a presentation that shows as well as tells and a peer mentor's exquisite listening is a land of enlightenment. Suddenly, obstacles you couldn't see around disappear, gaps you never noticed come into view and vanish in a blaze of awareness, and novel ways to engage your participants or new connections become clear and pull everything together. After your session, you'll tweak your presentation into a beauty of balance.

And all because you prepared yourself for your session and engaged in a dialogue with the colleague–friend who agreed to be your peer mentor.

Because most peer-mentoring relationships are reciprocal, meaning that you take turns peer mentoring one another's presentations, I'm assuming that you'll be a presenter at least half of the time in your relationship. So I wrote this section from the point of view of the presenter. Since few nurses have assistants, never mind mentors, having someone to help prepare your presentations can take some getting used to. Try it a few times and you'll find that peer mentoring is like spending a long weekend on an unspoiled island. If someone has to have a peer mentor, it might as well be you!

Because the peer-mentoring model is presenter driven, getting what you need and want is where the Pre-Session Questionnaire (PSQ) comes in. Completed prior to your pre-session, this questionnaire combines self-reflection questions with the specifics of what and how you're going to present. Using my peer-mentoring relationship with Karen as an example, this chapter reviews the first set of *Who* questions that allow you to reflect on yourself as a presenter and compare your style with that of your peer mentor. The following box shows how Karen's and my presenting styles compare.

My Response to *Who* Questions

My teaching style (Sage/Guide/Both): Guide on the Side

My future direction as a presenter: I want to develop my comfort with standing in the spotlight and responding to questions about my work in an even-handed manner that informs and impassions audiences.

My peer mentor's presenting style: Sage

Because ours is an ongoing peer-mentoring relationship, I knew Karen's presenting style without having to ask. If yours is a new peer-mentoring relationship or if you've never discussed your presenting styles before, wait until your pre-session to ask about your peer mentor's presenting style. When peer mentors don't know their styles, figure it out together by telling them the stories of Samantha, Tom, and Beth (see Chapter 12).

The few minutes it takes to retrieve your presenting style (Chapter 14) and your future direction as a presenter (Chapter 15) are worth it. By bringing this information to your pre-session, you and your peer mentor may find ways to capitalize on your presenting strengths and to make adjustments for your challenge, which *is* your future direction. Now it's your turn to respond to the *Who* questions in Jot Box 41-1.

Jot Box 41-1

Who **Questions**

Your teaching style (Sage/Guide/Both): _____

Your future direction as a presenter: _____

Your peer mentor's presenting style: _____

How was that for you to review your style and challenge/future direction?

The whole point in completing each PSQ section is generating a list of challenge questions to bring to your pre-session. As you can see from my response below, the challenge question in this *Who* section teams presenters and peer mentors in helping presenters manifest their future directions.

My Challenge Question

How will the mix of my peer mentor's and my presenting styles help me actualize my future direction as a presenter?

Sage-to-Guide Challenge: As a Sage, Karen calls me to develop more of a Sage-presenting style by encouraging me to take center stage and share my knowledge.

As you formulate your challenge question, keep in mind the advantages of having a peer mentor whose presenting is similar—communication is smooth, understanding instant—and having a peer mentor whose style is different. When you have a peer mentor whose style is different from your own, your differences challenge you to examine your assumptions and to stretch yourself as a presenter. Now it's your turn to complete the challenge question in Jot Box 41-2.

Jot Box 41-2

Your Challenge Question

How will the mix of your peer mentor's and your presenting styles help you actualize your future direction as a presenter?

_____

_____

_____

_____

The more you understand each other's aspirations as presenters and how your styles compare and contrast, the better your chances of having a meaningful peer-mentoring experience. The next two chapters help you develop challenge questions related to the *what* and *how* sections of your presentation.

TIP

It's a skill to ask for what you want so give yourself the permission to practice this skill with your peer mentor.

References

1. Costa, A. L., & Garmston, R. (1992). Cognitive coaching for peer reflection. *Journal of Supervision and Curricular Development, 5*(20), 15–19.
2. Heinrich, K. T., & Scherr, M. (1994, July–August). Peer mentoring for reflective teaching. *Nurse Educator, 19*(4), 36–41.

How to Prepare *What* Questions for Pre-Sessions with Peer Mentors

42

> *There are two ways to spread the light: to be the candle or the mirror that reflects it.*

Edith Wharton

Good news! Now that you've completed your Presentation Worksheet, you're ready to answer the *What* section in the PSQ. The first step is a simple transfer of information:

My Response to the *What* Section on the PSQ

My single idea/topic/focus/purpose? Designed to stimulate spirited dialogue, this interactive session engages participants in sharing stories about situations that stole their joy and strategizing responses that foster zestful academic environments.

My sweet-spot slant (title)? Joy-Stealing Games: What School Nurses Can Do to Stop the Game-Playing

(continues)

Who's my audience? How many? 80 to 100 school nurses

What's my desired audience response? To foster zestful school environments with zero-tolerance for such games

What's the length of my presentation? 50 minutes

Where & when is my presentation? 7:00 PM to 8:00 PM, October 26, 2006

What's the venue? Restaurant dining room

From my responses to the *What* section, you can tell that I was thinking ahead to my presentation to pinpoint areas of concern or anticipate problems. See how my responses translated into my two challenge questions below.

My *What* Challenge Questions

1. **Choreographic Challenge:** How do I engage participants when the group is seated at large round tables divided into two dining areas, one of which is adjacent to the kitchen?

2. **Biorhythm Challenge:** How do I keep my own and my participants' energy high when I'm not a night person and they've been working all day?

Now it's your turn. Feel free to scribble any concerns or potential problems noted as you transfer your information from your Presentation Worksheet to the PSQ on the following page.

Your Response to the *What* Section on the PSQ

My single idea/topic/focus/purpose? _____

My sweet-spot slant (title)? _____

Who's my audience? How many? _____

What's my desired audience response? _____

What's the length of my presentation? _____

Where and when is my presentation? _____

What's the venue? _____

What concerns came up for you as you were transferring your information into the PSQ *What* section? Are you wondering how I got from my worksheet items and concerns to my challenge questions? It's easy. As you transfer items to the *What* section, study them in the three ways described in Information Box 42-1 and you're sure to find a challenge question or two.

Information Box 42-1

How to Translate Items and Concerns into *What* Challenge Questions

1. **Item-by-item**. Make sure each item is complete. For example, when your slant/title does not contain both a descriptive and an emotive component, it's a "slant challenge."

2. **Compare items**. Look for misfits between items. For example, a misfit between your venue and your audience is a "choreographic challenge." A misfit between your purpose and your desired audience response is an "expectation challenge."

3. **Identify items that raise concerns for the presenter**. Look for any items that raise issues for you as a presenter. For example, it's a "biorhythm challenge" for me as a morning person to make evening presentations. As a shy person, presenting to an audience of 500 might be an "audience-size" challenge.

Have fun finding names for your challenges. Once you name them, challenges don't seem so scary anymore. Get ready to translate your items and concerns into challenge questions. Remember to include any questions or concerns related to your presentation packet or your PowerPoint slide display in your list of challenge questions as you complete Jot Box 42-1.

Jot Box 42-1

Your *What* Challenge Questions

_____

_____

_____

_____

_____

_____

_____

_____

_____

_____

By raising challenge questions in your pre-presentation session, you and your peer mentor will be able to address your concerns and strategize ways to handle potential problems.

TIP

Bring your challenge questions to your pre-session so you can answer them for yourself with the guidance of your peer mentor.

How to Prepare *How* Questions for Pre-Sessions with Peer Mentors

In the middle of difficulty lies opportunity.

Albert Einstein

The final section of the PSQ is devoted to *how* you're going to present. In this case, your Kolb-It Worksheet contains the information needed to complete the *How* section of the PSQ. This is how I completed the *How* section that I brought to my pre-presentation session with Karen.

My Response to the *How* Section

Session Title: Joy-Stealing Games: What School Nurses Can Do to Stop the Game-Playing

- **Concrete Experience:** Free-write your joy-stealing story/ Identify games
- **Reflective Observation:** What was that like for you to write your story?
- **Abstract Conceptualization:** Strategies to restore the zest
- **Active Experimentation:** The strategy I will use to restore the zest in my joy-stealing situation . . . (Free-write/Pair Share)

Transferring the information from my Kolb-It Worksheet reminded me of my dissatisfaction with my show-and-tell design. I knew it was weak, but it was the best I could do by myself. I needed Karen's input, both as a school nurse and as an educator familiar with Kolb's model. My *How* challenge question became, "How can I tailor the show-and-tell design and the theory to fit this school nurse audience?"

By bringing my design to our pre-session, Karen helped by reminding me that school nurses are doers who want to learn theory that they can apply to their practice tomorrow. This reminder, along with her questions about the original design, helped me to come up with the two-cycle design in which Karen opened the presentation session with her story about a school nurse who had her joy stolen by an administrator (Chapter 36).

Now it's your turn to transfer your Kolb-It Worksheet information to the PSQ *How* section in Jot Box 43-1.

Jot Box 43-1

Session Title: _____

Concrete Experience (CE): _____

Reflective Observation (RO): _____

Abstract Conceptualization (AC): _____

Active Experimentation (AE): _____

All challenge questions in the *How* section are design questions. Review the following possibilities when developing design challenge questions (see Information Box 43-1).

Information Box 43-1

How to Determine Design Challenge Questions

1. **Examine each learning activity:** How satisfied are you with each learning activity?
2. **Assess the flow:** How satisfied are you with the flow of one learning activity into another?
3. **Check for internal consistency:** How satisfied are you with how your slant is threaded throughout your Kolb-It design?

What design challenge questions emerged as you were transferring your information? (Use Jot Box 43-2.)

Jot Box 43-2

Your Design Challenge Questions

_____

_____

_____

_____

_____

_____

If you're satisfied with your design, you may not bring any *How* challenge questions to the pre-session. Don't be surprised, however, if design challenge questions emerge as you share your show-and-tell design with your peer mentor.

When these three sections—*Who, What,* and *How*—are put together, they form the one-page Pre-Session Questionnaire.

Pre-Session Questionnaire

What Questions

My presenting style (Sage/Guide/Both): _____

My peer mentor's presenting style: _____

My future direction as a presenter: _____

What Questions

What's my single idea/topic/focus/purpose? _____

Who's my audience? How many? _____

What's my desired audience response? _____

What's the length of my presentation? _____

Where and when is my presentation? _____

What's the venue? _____

What's my sweet-spot slant (title)? _____

How Questions

Concrete Experience: _____

Reflective Observation: _____

Abstract Conceptualization: _____

Active Experimentation: _____

The final step is listing your challenges from all three sections on one sheet, as I did in the following box.

My List of Challenge Questions for My Pre-Session

1. **Sage Challenge Question:** How can I develop my Sage-within by stepping into the spotlight during this presentation?
2. **Choreographic Challenge Question:** How do I engage participants when the group is seated at large round tables divided into two dining areas, one of which is adjacent to the kitchen?
3. **Biorhythm Challenge Question:** How do I keep my own and my participants' energy high for an evening session when I'm not a night person and they've been working all day?
4. **Design Challenge Question:** How can I tailor the show-and-tell design and the theory to fit this school-nurse audience?

Compile your own list of challenge questions in Jot Box 43-3.

Jot Box 43-3

Your List of Challenge Questions for Your Pre-Session

_____

_____

_____

_____

_____

_____

With your PSQ and your challenge questions completed, you're prepared for your pre-session.

TIP

Bring a beginner's mind to exploring your design for challenge questions.

How to Get the Most from Pre-Sessions with Peer Mentors

44

Imagine that you are a masterpiece unfolding every second of every day, a work of art taking form with every breath.

Thomas Crum

Now that you've completed your PSQ and your challenge questions, you've either sent them on to your peer mentor or you're bringing hard copies to your pre-session. The same goes for your presentation packet or PowerPoint slide display, should you wish to discuss either of these with your peer mentor. To keep pre-sessions on task, the peer mentor's questions are scripted and follow the sequence of the PSQ:

- Tell me about yourself as a presenter?
- Walk me through what and how you're going to present.
- What are your challenge questions?
- What help would you like from me during your presentation?
- What feedback would you like from me?

Each of the peer mentor's questions will be discussed separately.

Tell me about yourself as a presenter? Discussing your responses on the PSQ *Who* section will help your peer mentor get to know you as a presenter. A dialogue about your respective styles may help you capitalize on your strengths and move closer to your future direction.

Walk me through what and how you're going to present? Use your responses on the PSQ as a guide for describing the *What* and *How* of your presentation.

What are your challenge questions? Address each challenge question separately. Don't forget to include challenge questions related to your presentation packet and PowerPoint slide display.

What help would you like from me during your session? Peer mentors do not have to attend your presentation. When they do, this is the question they ask, because they can serve as an extra set of eyes and ears and hands.[1] Peer mentors can serve the following roles:

1. **Technical assistant:** Sets up audiovisual equipment (e.g. PowerPoint slide show, etc.).
2. **Rooter:** Is a smiling face in the audience.
3. **Logistics expert:** Handles choreographic challenges, distributes packets, collects evaluations, etc.
4. **Participant:** Has a speaking part in the presentation.

Karen is a great example of how a peer mentor can fulfill all four functions during a presentation. When she agreed to attend my after-dinner presentation, I asked that Karen be a smiling face in the audience, help with the choreographic challenges of presenting in a restaurant dining room, and collect participants' free-writes and evaluations. Going above and beyond, Karen drove us to the restaurant in her green, Volkswagen Bug so we could prepare on the way to and debrief after our presentation. Her parking angel nabbed us a spot right at the front door. Karen participated in the presentation by telling the story of a school nurse whose meeting with an administrator stole her joy. Beyond being a smiling face, Karen figured out where we should stand to be seen by all participants and collected free-writes and evaluations from audience-participants.

What feedback would you like from me? This is a question peer mentors ask when they plan to attend or to review a videotape/streaming video of your presentation. Asking for the feedback you want can take as much getting used to as having an assistant. Your request depends on a number of factors, including how seasoned a presenter you are, how comfortable you are with getting feedback on presentations, and what your trust level is with your peer mentor. When new to presenting, to peer mentoring, or to a particular peer mentor, it's fine to ask for only *positive* feedback (+). As your self-confidence grows along with the trust in your relationship, you'll probably ask for positives as well as suggestions for changes (+/-). If you like your feedback direct and clear, you may ask that your mentor address only that which needs to be fixed(-). As an experienced presenter who trusts my peer mentor to give me positive and constructively critical feedback, I asked Karen for the positives and negatives, both what she liked and what I could do differently. In my experience, nurse presenters respond best to the "compliment sandwich"—compliment, correct, compliment again (+/-/+).[2]

If peer mentoring is like a long weekend on an island, then asking for feedback is akin to giving instructions to a massage therapist. You tell your peer mentor how superficial or deep you want your feedback. Do you want to find out how many times you said "umm"? Or do you want your peer mentor to point out that more show and less tell will engage your audience even more?

After deciding *together* how your peer mentor will help you during the presentation (if your peer mentor is planning to attend your presentation) and what type of feedback you want after the presentation, you're good to go.

TIP

The best peer mentors listen, ask questions, and look for inconsistencies.

References

1. Heinrich, K. T., & Scherr, M. (1994, July/August). Peer mentoring for reflective teaching. *Nurse Education, 19*(4), 36–41.
2. Challoner, K. (2006, December). The compliment sandwich. *O Magazine.*

How to Prepare for Post-Sessions with Peer Mentors

45

Assessment will gradually become an integral part of every [presenter's] reflective practice.

P. T. Ewell

Now that your presentation is over, give yourself a pat on the back. You've worked hard to prepare your session with input from your peer mentor. Although at this point you may just want to let down and relax, it's not yet time. Actually, this is a fun part, because you get to reflect on your presentation and find out how your audience-participants responded. By now, it won't surprise you that a couple of worksheets are involved. You can complete these in any order you wish. I'm sharing them in the order I complete them—the What Worked & Future Changes Worksheet and the Audience Feedback Worksheet. The best time to complete these worksheets is as soon after your presentation as possible. Once you do, you'll be ready for your post-session.

Using my reflections on the presentation to the school-nurse group, you can see my What Worked & Future Changes Worksheet.

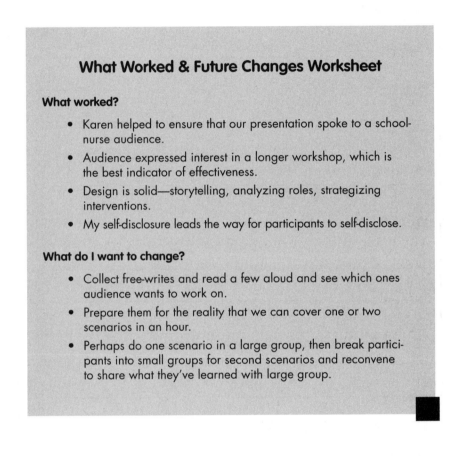

What Worked & Future Changes Worksheet

What worked?

- Karen helped to ensure that our presentation spoke to a school-nurse audience.
- Audience expressed interest in a longer workshop, which is the best indicator of effectiveness.
- Design is solid—storytelling, analyzing roles, strategizing interventions.
- My self-disclosure leads the way for participants to self-disclose.

What do I want to change?

- Collect free-writes and read a few aloud and see which ones audience wants to work on.
- Prepare them for the reality that we can cover one or two scenarios in an hour.
- Perhaps do one scenario in a large group, then break participants into small groups for second scenarios and reconvene to share what they've learned with large group.

Use the following blank What Worked & Future Changes Worksheet after your next presentation.

What Worked & Future Changes Worksheet

What worked?

_____

_____

_____

_____

_____

What do you want to change?

_____

_____

_____

_____

_____

As Carl Jung once said of dreams, not taking audience feedback into account is like leaving a letter from a friend unopened.[1] As you may remember from Chapter 38, my evaluation forms ask participants to respond to three items: appreciations, critiques, and affirmations. After reading all the responses from the school-nurse audience, I collated their responses. To collate is to group audience participants' responses by item. After typing in all the responses to each question, I reviewed them. When there was repetition, I chose the most descriptive and deleted the redundant comments. To see how it feels to read appreciations and critiques, read this feedback from my audience as if it came from a presentation you gave.

Collation of Audience Feedback Results

Joy-Stealing: How School Nurses Can Stop the Game-Playing
Association of CT School Nurses
October 26, 2006
N = 31/117 (33%)

Appreciation:

Joy-stealers . . . yes, they exist. I liked that you understood what school nurses deal with.

Audience participation made us realize that we all have the same day-to-day struggles.

Not what we expected.

Very empowering design. Liked the real-life stories and the opportunity to analyze and strategize. It was purposeful and different than the usual bitch and moan.

Good tools for life's bumps. We all need strategies to deal with joy-stealers.

Interactive, intuitive speaker. Continue working your magic with school nurses and help us find our true voices.

Pleasurable surroundings.

This should be a whole day workshop, think about that please.

Critique:

I would have liked to hear more stories and more brainstorming.

Would rather have had situations submitted beforehand and facilitator choose a good one.

I felt that this lecture stated the obvious. The pace could be picked up also.

More sharing in small groups (2).

Different seating. Side bar conversations and noise from the kitchen distracting.

How was it for you to read these comments? If you're like me, reading the positive comments felt good because they were affirming. That's why I put the "good stuff" up front. I find it easier to take in participants' critiques after reading the accolades.

I collate the responses to the final item—affirmations—to assess how effective a presentation is in meeting my purpose for presenting, which, in this case, is to educate and move school nurse participants to action. As you can see, I matched the language in their affirmations with these two purposes.

Match Audience Affirmations to Purpose

Educate, Learning
> I am an ally to myself.
> I appreciate the many allies in my life.

Motivate, Move to Action
> No more stewing. I figure out solutions, not just discuss problems.
> I reach out and ask for help because many heads are helpful.
> I decide on an intervention and practice it beforehand.
> I deal with the problem upfront without anger.
> I stand up for myself even when I'm frightened about doing so.

Behavioral Objective:
> After this workshop, participants will initiate a dialogue about how school nurses can foster zestful school environments with zero-tolerance for joy-stealing games.

Not only was there a match between participants' affirmations and purposes, but their affirmations confirmed that the behavioral objective written into the presentation packet had been met.

When reviewing audience-participants' feedback, I've found three strategies to be useful:

1. **Set a still point.** Centering myself before I read evaluations allows me to accept both appreciations and critiques with equanimity.
2. **Stay the decider.** Deciding which feedback to use or discard in refining future offerings is my responsibility as a presenter. Do bring questions or concerns raised by feedback to your post-session so they can be discussed with your peer mentor.

3. **Be consistent.** Find an evaluation form that fits, stick with it and collate your audience feedback the same way after every presentation.

Make it a practice, after each learning episode, to collate your evaluation feedback. If you use a presentation evaluation format that's different than mine, you'll need to make up a format for your own Audience Feedback Sheet.

TIP
Raise your audience awareness quotient by determining what worked and what to change and collating audience feedback after every presentation.

References

1. Jung, C. G. (1973). *Memories, dreams, reflections.* New York: Pantheon Books.

How to Make the Most of Post-Sessions with Peer Mentors

46

*Anything or anyone that does not bring
you alive is too small for you.*

David Whyte

When we got into Karen's Beetle to drive home following the presentation, the first thing I said was, "So what did you think of my presentation?" As a good peer mentor, even though it frustrates me every time she does it, Karen turned the question back to me by asking, "What did *you* like about your presentation?" See why I asked her to be my peer mentor?

Just as questions for the pre-presentation session are scripted, peer mentors use four scripted questions to guide presenters' reflections during the post-presentation session.[1]

1. What did you like about your presentation?
2. What would you change?
3. Would you like to hear my feedback?
4. How could I be a better peer mentor for you?

When your peer mentor attends your presentation, you can answer some of these questions together. Karen and I used our drive home to debrief. I would recommend that, whether your peer mentor attends your presentation or not, you also schedule a mutually convenient hour for a post-presentation session within a week of your presentation. A week allows just enough time to get some distance and not too much to forget the details. It also gives you enough time to complete your What Worked & Future Changes Worksheet and collate audience feedback. Let's discuss each of the peer-mentoring questions in order.

What did you like about your presentation? When, like Karen, peer mentors keep the spotlight on the positive, you'll find yourself with a long list of likes that can surprise you. Combining my list of *what worked* with the *audience appreciations* I collated, the following is my list of likes:

- Karen's input during our pre-session relieved my pre-session jitters about making this presentation relevant to school nurses.
- Karen's help with figuring out choreographic challenges like where we should stand so we could be seen and heard by the entire audience.
- The story Karen told gave them such a great example of joy-stealing roles.
- The set up of the free-write that involved asking audience participants to stay quiet and to keep their pens moving was effective.
- The school nurse participant who shared her joy-stealing story and all the ideas she got from her colleagues for dealing with her situation.
- The number of strategies for negotiating joy-stealing situations that audience generated from a single example.
- There was just the right amount of theory.
- Participants' free-writes revealed 10 steps for dealing with joy-stealing situations.

What would you change about your presentation? Based on my list of *future changes* and *audience critiques*, this is what I'd do differently:

- Give audience 2 minutes to share what it was like to write their joy-stealing story with the person sitting next to them. Then everyone would have the opportunity to share without feeling like they had to reveal the details of their joy-stealing story.
- Orchestrate the choreographic challenge of collecting audience free-writes by designating a representative from each table to gather them and give them to Karen.

Notice how short the list of future changes is compared with my list of likes.

Would you like my feedback? Now it's your peer mentor's turn to give you feedback. Karen's feedback addressed the requests I made during our pre-session to tell me everything she liked and everything she would change about my presentation. Because this is a presenter-driven model, your peer mentor gives you only the feedback that you asked for. That's why it's important to ask for the feedback you want in your pre-session. Karen's feedback on my session was as follows:

- I liked how you kept the pace energetic and engaging so everyone was involved, which was no small task given that we were in a restaurant dining room.
- The presentation was effective because the stories really did show audience participants what joy-stealing games look like, which allowed you to share the theory with them.
- Your use of self-disclosure was very effective, like when you shared how difficult it is to be assertive at times.

How could I be a better peer mentor for you? The final question turns the tables as peer mentors ask presenters how to improve their peer-mentoring skills. Here's what I said when Karen asked how she could be a better peer mentor:

- You were a great peer mentor. Not only did you help make sure that this presentation spoke to school nurses, you shared a story that really resonated with the crowd.
- It was such a comfort to have you there during the presentation and to have you attend to logistics like passing out the handouts and collecting the free-writes.
- As a Sage, you always challenge me to own my inner-Sage by stepping into the spotlight.

Peer-mentoring relationships are intended to be ongoing, so if you have suggestions for your peer mentor sharing them in an honest discussion will enhance your peer-mentoring experience the next time.

In truth, post-sessions are often a time to celebrate your accomplishment with your peer mentor. So enjoy! After your session, file your What Worked and Future Changes Worksheet and Audience Feedback Sheet, along with a summary list of changes gleaned during your post-session and your presentation packet, in a folder labeled with the name of your presentation. Then, when you get the opportunity to give a presentation on a similar topic in the future, you've got the feedback from three sources—yourself, your audience, and your peer mentor—to guide your revisions.

And finally, don't forget to express your gratitude to your colleague–friend for acting as your peer mentor. I write a formal letter of appreciation on my company letterhead that specifies the title, date, and place of the presentation and the peer mentor's contributions along with my thanks for his or her generous sharing of time, expertise, and energy.

Now that you've prepared for both the pre- and post-session, you'll be able to reflect on future presentations whether you have the luxury of a peer mentor or not. That's why peer mentoring is a gift that keeps on giving for the whole of your professional career.

TIP

Be a reflective presenter! Review your likes and changes after every presentation.

References

1. Costa, A. L., & Garmston, R. (1992). Cognitive coaching for peer reflection. *Journal of Supervision and Curricular Development, 5*(20), 15–19.

Why a Storytelling Chapter?

47

*You gain strength, courage, and confidence
by every experience in which you really
stop to look fear in the face.*

Eleanor Roosevelt

What's the best way to get a feel for what it's like to present? Work-sheets and questionnaires are all well and good, but they can't give you pre-presentation jitters; that night-before dream about presenting with half of your business suit missing; the humility that comes over you as you stand before a group that's gathered together to listen to you; the exhilaration when the show's over and you're still alive; the joys and stings from reading audience comments; or the intensity of rehashing the highs and lows with your peer mentor.

Just this morning I was thinking how it's really like reading *Gourmet* or *Cooking Light*. No matter how beautiful the photographs or how deli-cious sounding the ingredient list, there's not a picture or a word that can convey what an oatmeal cookie with white-chocolate-chips and cranberries smells like straight out of the oven. For that you need your smell-agination. So, too, with presenting. The three-dimensional, real-life experience is so much more delectable than the one-dimensional planning steps can convey.

In baking terminology, this section needs the puff that only baking powder can give.[1] The only way to breathe dimensionality into a flat page is to engage imaginations through storytelling. So that's why this section closes with Diana Mixon and Kelley Connor's story of their collaboration on a poster presentation. Peeking over their capable shoulders, you'll learn as much from their mistakes as from what they did well. They'll show you how to write a proposal that sells your idea, tells you which fonts to use on PowerPoint slides, and reminds you to coordinate your outfit with the colors in your poster. After reading their chapter, you'll never leave home without Velcro.

Just when I was playing with that baking analogy, I came across an article in *The New Yorker* about the dimensional challenge faced by those who write about food. To get you in the mood for a show-and-tell chapter that puffs three dimensions into the process of presenting a poster, I'll leave you with this thought:

> The act of reading is always a matter of a task begun as much as of a message understood, something that begins on a flat surface, counter or page, and then gets stirred and chopped and blended until what we make, in the end is a dish, or story, all our own.[2]

As you read the next chapter, find a way, whether you stir, chop, or blend the message, to make Diana and Kelley's story your own.

References

1. Strynkowski, B. (2007, May). Soda spreads, powder puffs. Ask Chef Billy. *Cooking Light,* 32.
2. Gopnik, A. (2007, April 9). Cooked books. Readings. *The New Yorker Magazine,* 85.

How to Make Sure Your Poster Is Worth a Thousand Words

48

Diana Mixon, RN, MSN and Kelley Connor, RNC, MS

Simplicity is the ultimate sophistication.

Leonardo da Vinci

Gwen and Jill arrive 30 minutes before the first poster session at a national conference. Gwen is carrying the cardboard tube that contains their 4-by-6-foot laminated poster. Jill is in charge of the portable DVD that accompanies the poster presentation. The first thing they notice is that everyone else has free-standing posters, and there are no electrical outlets to be found. What Gwen and Jill did not notice in the instructions that accompanied the acceptance letter was that posters were to be free-standing; if presenters brought their own extension cords, they could use one of the few electrical outlets. Gwen and Jill are left to improvise. Before you find out what they did, write about what you would do (see Jot Box 48-1).

Here's how Jill and Gwen handled the situation. Jill obtained a couple of cardboard boxes from one of the hotel's restaurants to construct a make-shift support. Taping the poster to the cardboard backing kept the poster upright, but the ends kept curling because the tape didn't stick very well. With repeated tape reinforcement, they managed. The DVD player's battery needed to be charged after every hour of use, so they took turns recharging it.

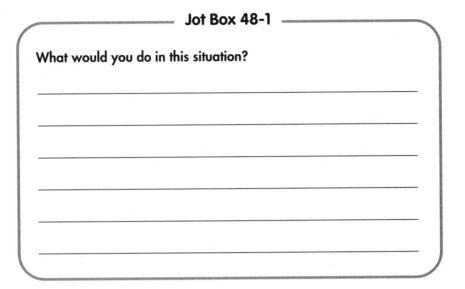

Gwen and Jill were able to present their information, but the experience wasn't what they expected. We (Diana and Kelley) decided to tell you our story to help you avoid having an experience like Gwen and Jill's. In this chapter, we share the step-by-step process for finding venues, creating abstracts for professional conferences, and developing and displaying posters. You'll read how our poster presentation became an unexpected networking opportunity that allowed us to discuss our project informally with almost 500 conference participants. In addition to making valuable professional connections, these dialogues expanded our perspective, gave us exhilarating ideas for future ventures, and laid the groundwork for writing this chapter.

After reading about our experience, you'll know how to create a poster that's worth a thousand words! In fact, you've already learned an invaluable lesson from Gwen and Jill's story. It's important to follow directions whether you're writing a proposal/abstract or standing by your poster ready to answer questions at times specified by conference conveners.

Deciding To Present Our Project

Before joining the Boise State University faculty last year, Kelley was a clinician and staff development educator. Diana is a tenured nurse educator, as well as Kelley's faculty mentor. In response to a community need and to meet student objectives for a clinical course, we, along with two other faculty colleagues, designed and implemented a successful health fair project for nursing students. We wanted to work smart by turning this teaching-learning activity into a presentation. The question was how. Although we knew it was our professional responsibility to share our project with other educator colleagues, the thought of a formal "presentation" to a large group was intimidating. To be honest, a poster presentation seemed like the least-threatening way to share our findings. At the same time, this experience would give Kelley credit for a presentation at a national conference for her promotion and tenure dossier. In every sense, this project would become a true partnership; Kelley's technology skills augmenting Diana's previous experiences with presenting posters.

Finding a Venue

After deciding to present a poster, we needed to find a place to present. We considered surfing the Internet for events or conferences sponsored by local health-care agencies, such as hospitals or health departments. We also thought about conferences sponsored by universities, such as the Drexel University Nursing Education Institute, professional organizations, such as the Association of Women's Health, Obstetric, and Neonatal Nurses (AWHONN) and the Association of Nurses in AIDS Care (ANAC), or private textbook companies, such as Mosby. In the end, it was a personal connection that helped make our venue decision.

Because ours was an education-related project, we were looking for an education conference with a theme that fit our topic. In reviewing the flyer for Mosby's Faculty Development Institute, we noticed that one of the conference objectives was to ". . . explain strategies faculty can implement for career development and mobility." One of our colleagues, Dr. Cynthia Clark, was a conference coordinator. When we approached Cindy with our idea, she thought a poster presentation was a great idea. When we reviewed the presentation topics, we saw a presenter's name we recognized, Kathleen Heinrich. Kathy had facilitated a faculty development workshop on presenting and publishing for our faculty group in January 2006. After that workshop, she peer edited a manuscript for Diana and her co-authors that was accepted for publication. When we e-mailed Kathy to ask her opinion, she agreed that our topic was a good fit with the conference's theme—Beyond the Box: Meeting the Challenges of Being a Nurse Educator Today. Unbeknownst to us, our reaching out to Kathy was initiating a new collaboration.

After selecting Mosby's Teaching Institute as a venue, we reviewed the "Call for Posters." The instructions specified the length of the abstract, how to submit the document, and the target date for notification of acceptance. The acceptance notification would include the information about the space allotted for the poster, the size of the poster, whether the poster needed to be free-standing, and available amenities, such as easels and electrical outlets.

We decided not to register for the conference or secure hotel rooms until we knew that our proposal had been accepted. After we received notification, we realized that the poster acceptance date was after the due date for the early registration rate and lower room rates. We were able to negotiate the early conference registration rate, but the hotel would not agree to the conference room rate. Our hotel room ended up costing us $100 more per night! A second lesson learned—check the dates for registration and acceptance of posters to ensure you can take advantage of reduced rates!

Composing Our Proposal Abstract

Mosby's only stipulation was that the proposal abstract be no longer than one page. Because we were vague about what information to include, we searched the Internet for formats and reviewed the poster abstracts our colleagues had written. In the process we discovered that an abstract should *sell* our work. Our proposal abstract ended up including the following headings.[1]

1. Title
2. Authors
3. Affiliation
4. Purpose and Rationale of Work
5. Description of the Problem
6. Approach to Solving the Problem
7. Answer to the Problem
8. Implications of the Answer
9. References

You can read the proposal that sold our project to the Mosby conference conveners in the following box.

Proposal

Title: Spinning the Scholarship of Teaching and Learning into Research

Co-Presenters: Kelley Connor, R.N.C., M.S., Diana Mixon, R.N., M.S.N, Ginny Gilbert, R.N., M.S.N, Leonie Sutherland, R.N., PhD

Institution: Boise State University, Boise, Idaho

Purpose and Rationale: Throughout academia, nursing educators are challenged to prepare graduates who can perform effectively in complex healthcare environments. Simultaneously, educators are charged with advancing the profession of nursing through programs of research. An established method to accomplish these goals is through the Scholarship of Teaching and Learning (SoTL). Using the SoTL framework, nurse educators can transform the programs and projects employed in education and turn them into scholarly activities.

Description of Project: A logic model was developed to evaluate the outcomes of a community-based clinical experience involving students in third and forth semesters of a baccalaureate nursing program. The model provides a map for faculty identifying key evaluation points to measure student learning. Using these points, research and evaluative questions can be developed to determine outcomes for individual and overall program goals. For example, one of the first questions we want to explore is: What are the perceptions of beginning nursing students regarding their ability to present health information to a group of employees at the Idaho Department of Health and Welfare? This question links the activity of conducting a health fair with the outcome of the students' ability to teach.

Conclusion: The logic model will provide various options for continued evaluation leading to an ongoing program of collaborative faculty/student research. Designed by four faculty at a metropolitan university of distinction in the Northwest, the logic model illustrates how the SoTL can be used as a framework to enhance scholarly achievement.

References:
Ellermann, C. R., Kataoka-Yahiro, M. R., & Wong, L. C. (2006). Logic models used to enhance critical thinking. *Journal of Nursing Education, 45*(6), 220–227.
Heinrich, K. T. (2005, February 15). Do what savy educators do: Turn your teaching into scholarship. NLN Audio-web seminar.
Heinrich, K. T. (2006, January 12). With eyes a'glitter: From passionate teacher to passionate scholar. Boise State University Department of Nursing, Boise, ID.
Heinrich, K. T., & Neese, R. (2004). Assessing the ineffable: The challenge for nursing education. *Annual Review of Nursing Education.* Vol. 2. New York: Springer Publications, 71–88.

Designing the Poster

Once we received confirmation that our poster proposal had been accepted, we took ourselves to lunch to celebrate. From there, we reviewed our proposal and the instructions in the acceptance letter. Mosby's acceptance information included the size of both the poster and the table, which in this case was 8 by 4 feet, and indicated that posters were to be free-standing with limited access to electrical connections.

Although these guidelines formed the basis for our poster design, at this point we were unsure about how to put our poster together. Cost was an issue, so we considered several options before making a final decision. Our institution, as do others, offers a set amount of funding for poster preparation. Some facilities have an instructional technology or instructional design department to assist with design. When these resources are unavailable, commercial graphic arts companies will design posters for you or you can "do it yourself." Using an online search engine, we found a plethora of poster design articles, online courses, online templates, and instructional sites, so we felt adequately equipped to tackle the design work ourselves.

When we were thinking about poster design, we considered using a large single sheet that could be rolled up for transport. This form of poster is printed on a special machine, usually found in an instructional design department. The sheets can be as large as 8 by 4 feet, and they look like a poster one would buy at the mall. We realized that this format would not be free-standing and our department's sturdy cylindrical carrying case was awkward to transport. We decided to develop a smaller poster that could be made with PowerPoint slides or another slide-based presentation software product in which each slide is printed on 8 1/2 by 11-inch paper. Such slides can be matted on colored paper or attached to foam backing. Either of these formats can be laminated to preserve the slide. Slides are easy to transport and can be affixed easily to a poster display board. We decided on laminated slides attached to foam backing. We attached the slides to a 3-foot by 4-foot trifold display board with Velcro.

Using our university's instructional design department, we were able to produce our poster slides and the synopsis handouts for less than $150.00. Because our department already had a 3-foot by 4-foot free-standing trifold stand to display the slides, this was not included in the cost.

Attracting Attention to Our Poster

We wanted to make a visual impact with our poster. Given that we might not be present when our poster was viewed, our poster had to be self-explanatory and concise in relaying outcomes and achievements.[2] In other words, it would need to attract attention and "stand on its own" in terms of the viewer being able to clearly discern content. To keep the poster readable, we used white space to organize the information. From our reading, we learned that posters can flow in one of two ways, by columns or by rows. Although both schemes work, gravity naturally pulls the eyes from top to bottom and then left to right. When using rows, viewers usually need to stop and turn their head to read the content of the poster.[2] With this in mind, our poster had three columns with three slides in the first two columns and four slides in the third column. The proposal abstract you just read was our 10th slide.

For us, the beauty of computerized formatting is that we could play with several layouts to see which display provided the most clarity for our information. We immediately noticed that headings helped viewers find the information they needed to understand our topic. Because our poster displays a research project, we used the same headings that appeared in our proposal abstract: purpose, problem, design, results, and conclusion.[3]

Successful posters are a visually pleasing arrangement of graphics, text, and color. The 10 guidelines we followed ensured that our poster was as appealing as it was easy to read:[2,3]

1. Keep it simple. Use two or three colors.
2. Make the poster easy to read. Dark letters on a light background are the easiest to read.
3. Avoid bright colors. Although they attract attention, they tend to tire the eyes.
4. Make the title stand out. The poster title should be the first thing a viewer sees.
5. Make the font larger for headings than for the text.
6. Use a simple font for text (e.g. Times New Roman) at a minimum size of 24 point or larger. Test the font size for readability. If all printed material can be seen from a distance of 3 to 6 feet away, your poster font passes the test.
7. Limit text to blocks of no more that 50 to 70 words.

8. When using graphs, focus on relationships, not specific data. A poster graph should provide a visual synopsis of relationships between variables. Convey the findings in a concise way; keep your graphs simple and uncluttered. Eliminate grid lines, markers, and legends. As an example, see Figure 48-1, which shows a graph depicting the frequency of hand washing and the decline of infection rates.

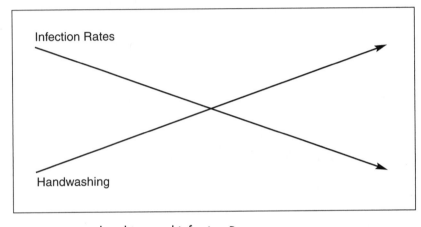

FIGURE 48-1   Handwashing and Infection Rates

9. Balance the arrangement of graphics and text.
10. Include contact information. The viewer should have all the contact information needed to contact you.

Note that titles attract attention when the slant is snazzy, the font is the largest on the poster, and they are in the form of a banner. Boise State University had just won the 2007 Fiesta Bowl, so we choose to put "Boise State University, Department of Nursing" in 48-point font on our banner, which is a 16-by-6-inch rectangle clipped to the top of the display board. Some of the conference attendees stopped by our poster just to discuss the football game. The point is that the banner should "hook" the viewers. Our poster title, in 44-point font, "Spinning the Scholarship of Teaching and Learning into Research," was on the first slide in the middle column, and it was positioned higher on the board than the two slides on either side of it.

To show you what we mean, one of our poster's slides is reproduced in Figure 48-2.

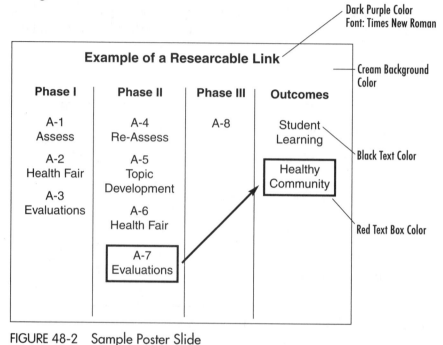

FIGURE 48-2   Sample Poster Slide

Ask Colleagues to Preview Your Poster

We made a mock poster our last step before finalizing the design. As a final check, we enlisted several colleagues to review our mock poster by answering the following questions:

1. Is the design appealing and easy to read?
2. Does the poster illustrate our abstract?
3. Is all the printing in the same font unless the font is being used to designate different sections or identify concepts?
4. Are all words spelled correctly? Is the text grammatically correct?
5. Is our contact information complete and easily located?

We used PowerPoint to make each slide. When we made copies of the slides, some of the text changed to another font, font sizing changed, and spacing changed. Luckily we had plenty of time to review the slides and make corrections. Although we thought our poster was complete, based on our colleagues' feedback we made changes that improved the content and the readability of our final product.

Technical Considerations

When it comes to posters, two sets of details must be considered: design and display. To prevent an on-site Gwen-and-Jill situation, ask yourself the same design questions that we asked ourselves at home:

1. Will you need a special easel?
2. How will you attach the poster to the board? Tape, Velcro, tacks?
3. What's your backup plan if the attaching medium doesn't hold?

Surprises are inevitable—the sticky tape that worked great in your office may lose its stick in the humidity of the conference room. We erred on the side of caution and came prepared with self-adhesive Velcro, a stapler, extra staples, paperclips, Scotch tape, safety pins, needle and thread, and Gorilla tape all packed in a box with our foam-backed slides.

To attract participants to our poster, as well as to enhance networking opportunities during and following the conference, we added the following special touches to our display:

- We supplied a two-sided take-away handout that summarized our poster. We included the abstract on one side and six of our PowerPoint slides on the other.
- We offered candy in colors that complemented those in our poster.
- We supplied business cards with our contact information, stapling them to our handout so attendees would have all of our information in one place when they got home.

Once we decided on our design and covered last-minute display details, it was time to make travel arrangements for our poster. Whether carting the poster down the hall, across town, or onto a plane, it's necessary to pack materials so they aren't damaged in transit. Because we were flying, we knew that some airlines charge extra for packages that are bulky or oversized. To avoid surprises, we called ahead and asked about size limitations. To transport our poster, we put tissues between the foam-backed slides, slid them into a box, included our extra supplies, and packed them into one of our suitcases. Even though airport security opened the transport box in the suitcase and rearranged the contents, the individual slides came through without scratches. The display board had its own carrying case that traveled with our luggage.

Presenting Our Poster

After we checked in for the pre-conference, we started to walk away because the first poster session didn't start until the next day. When we overheard the host mention that poster presenters could set up ahead of time, we stopped to clarify the time allocated for poster setup as well as the times we were required to be in attendance. We were told that time would be available later that afternoon for poster setup. Although some conferences allocate specific display areas, this conference gave poster presenters a choice as to where to setup their posters. We chose a place at the end of an aisle so we could have more space.

On the day of the presentation we wore professional clothing that matched the black, red, and white colors in our poster. We have since learned about research that suggests that more conference participants stop to view the posters of presenters who wear coordinating, rather than contrasting, colors.[4] During the poster sessions, Diana stood on one side facing the flow of traffic, Kelley stood on the opposite side. Diana had many more participants stop and talk to her about the poster than did Kelley. Another lesson learned—put the presenter who likes to talk more facing the traffic flow. Only kidding! We did spend more time than was required standing by our poster because we found talking with participants and clarifying their questions so stimulating. Not to mention that we might have missed a publishing opportunity if we weren't standing next to our poster. Kathy, when she saw our poster, said it was one of the best at the conference. She so appreciated the innovativeness of our project, the eye appeal of our display, and the clarity of our message that she asked us to "dare to share" our approach to presenting posters in this book chapter.

The only downside to spending so much time tending our own poster presentation was that we missed or were late to some of the sessions we wanted to attend because we lost track of time. A benefit of having co-presenters is that when one is attending a session, the other can cover the poster presentation. So another lesson is to include the sessions you want to attend in your schedule and allow yourself the time needed to get to session rooms with minutes to spare.

Use Posters to Share What You Do

If the poster fairy forced us to give you eight tips for sharing what you do in poster presentations, they would be:

1. Decide if your project lends itself to a visual art form such as a poster presentation.
2. Select a conference with a theme that fits your project.
3. Follow the poster guidelines from the conference conveners to guide your design.
4. Keep the design simple.
5. Make all printed text readable at 3 to 6 foot distances.
6. Ask your colleagues to preview your poster presentation.
7. Wear clothing that complements the colors in your poster.
8. Create a one-page handout that summarizes your work with your contact information.

Now that you're so well-prepared, you can relax and enjoy the conference! This will free you up to be more open to the new collaborations and professional opportunities that come from taking the dare to present what you do.

TIP
Combine simplicity, an artful display using white space, and attention to detail for a poster that's worth a thousand words!

References

1. Koopman, P. (1997). *How to write an abstract.* Retrieved August 20, 2007, from http://www.ece.cmu.edu/~koopman/essays/abstract.html
2. Larive, C. K., & Bulska, E. (2006). Tips for effective poster presentations. *Analytical and Bioanalytical Chemistry, 38*(5), 1618–2650.

3. Hess, G., Tosney, K., & Liegel, L. (2004). *Creating effective poster presentations: An effective poster.* Retrieved August 20, 2007, from http://www.ncsu.edu/project/posters

4. Moule, P., Judd, M., & Girot, E. (1998). The poster presentation: What value to the teaching and assessment of research in pre- and post-registration nursing courses? *Nurse Education Today, 18*(3), 237–242.

Conclusion: Commit to Presenting What You Do

49

As we give fully, unafraid to let others know the truth about ourselves, we receive unexpected rewards from unexpected sources.

Helene Lerner-Robbins

Congratulations! By taking it one step at a time, you've learned more about yourself as a presenter. You've also learned what to present, who to choose as a peer mentor, when to negotiate mindful relationships with co-presenters, and how to prepare for peer-mentoring sessions. After all that, are you feeling ready to present what you do? Before you answer, let's read your nurse companions' responses to the free-write question "I commit to presenting what I do by . . ."

Keri wrote:

> submitting a proposal for a poster presentation to a national nurse practitioner conference that compares excerpts from my journal about my "first year" experiences as a nurse practitioner with the findings from my thesis.

Betty's free-write reads:

> submitting a proposal to our Nurse's Day Hospital Planning Committee to facilitate a session on the ways we as nurses can

support each other to present and publish what we do. I've even got a peer mentor in mind if, wait a minute—I want to think positive so let me back up and say this the way I mean it. I've got a peer mentor lined up for *when* my proposal gets accepted.

Justin writes:

> . . . starting with a poster presentation at the National Student Nurses' Association. That way I'll organize my ideas and share our "Men in Nursing" initiative with lots of colleagues in a low-stress venue. Who knows, maybe someone who sees my poster will ask me to write that article I've wanted to publish.

Committing by submitting. That's what Keri, Betty, and Justin are doing by turning their everyday experiences into presentation proposals. To help you to respond to this free-write, scan the following 15 Powerful Presenting Practices in Information Box 49-1.

Information Box 49-1

Powerful Presenting Practices

1. Capitalize on your presenting style.
2. Identify your future direction as a presenter.
3. Don your presenter's persona.
4. Increase your audience awareness.
5. Get physical with your still point.
6. Select an eye-glittering idea.
7. Design a project timeline.
8. Complete a Presentation Worksheet.
9. Kolb your presentation.
10. Develop a PowerPoint display.
11. Create a presentation packet.
12. Choose your peer mentor well.
13. Negotiate mindful relationships with co-presenters.
14. Prepare challenge questions for your pre-session.
15. Refine presentations with feedback from you, your audience, and your peer mentor.

Take a minute to write your response in Jot Box 49-1.

Jot Box 49-1

I commit to presenting what I do by . . .

_____

_____

_____

_____

_____

_____

_____

_____

Did you or didn't you? Commit yourself, that is, to the next step. Whatever you wrote, your response tells you how close you are to taking the dare to present what you do.

When you embark on your next presentation project, use the checklist in Information Box 49-2 to ensure that your presentation is all that you want it to be.

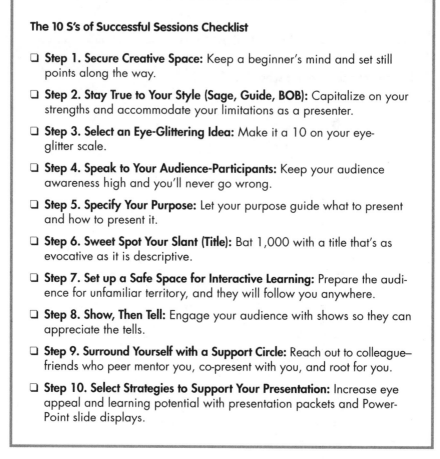

Information Box 49-2

The 10 S's of Successful Sessions Checklist

❑ **Step 1. Secure Creative Space:** Keep a beginner's mind and set still points along the way.

❑ **Step 2. Stay True to Your Style (Sage, Guide, BOB):** Capitalize on your strengths and accommodate your limitations as a presenter.

❑ **Step 3. Select an Eye-Glittering Idea:** Make it a 10 on your eye-glitter scale.

❑ **Step 4. Speak to Your Audience-Participants:** Keep your audience awareness high and you'll never go wrong.

❑ **Step 5. Specify Your Purpose:** Let your purpose guide what to present and how to present it.

❑ **Step 6. Sweet Spot Your Slant (Title):** Bat 1,000 with a title that's as evocative as it is descriptive.

❑ **Step 7. Set up a Safe Space for Interactive Learning:** Prepare the audience for unfamiliar territory, and they will follow you anywhere.

❑ **Step 8. Show, Then Tell:** Engage your audience with shows so they can appreciate the tells.

❑ **Step 9. Surround Yourself with a Support Circle:** Reach out to colleague–friends who peer mentor you, co-present with you, and root for you.

❑ **Step 10. Select Strategies to Support Your Presentation:** Increase eye appeal and learning potential with presentation packets and Power-Point slide displays.

TIP
Commitment is an essential step in presenting what you do

Small Steps to Write About What You Do

3

Introduction: Why Do Nurse Authors Get Addicted to Writing?

Notice who the author is in the top right corner! It took me a year to get my manuscript published but it was well worth it! Thank you for all your inspiration! I will send you a clear, printed copy as soon as I get them but I couldn't wait to show you!

Lisa Malchiodi

Even if there weren't exclamation points at the end of each sentence, every letter in Lisa's e-mail message vibrates with excitement. After taking the "Writing for Publication" workshop during her graduate program and presenting a poster on the topic, it would take Lisa a year of patience and perseverance to get her article on thyroid storm published. It used to be that academic nurses were the only ones who needed to publish. With hospitals pursuing magnet status, clinicians like Lisa are being encouraged to write about what they do. As publishing becomes an expectation for more nurses, a "nice to do" is becoming a "must do." This section can make writing a "want to do" for you.

It doesn't matter if publishing is a personal goal or if your job depends on it, once you see your name in print, you'll be hooked.

Rather than feeling finished after you've presented, you'll learn to "work smart" by funneling the positive energy and constructive feedback from your audiences into writing about what you do. As you shift to a work-smart perspective, you'll find your preferred writing style; learn how to locate the best home for your manuscript; write to your readers to elicit the response you're seeking; query editors; complete Publication Worksheets; decide if you're a free-writer, mind-mapper, or outliner; chunk your outline into 15 minute writing sessions; and transform your "shitty first draft" into a manuscript with the help of peer editors. In the process, you'll develop the four qualities authors need to complete writing projects: Dreamer (gathering ideas); Designer (organizing ideas); Builder (development and detail); and Inspector (refinement).[1]

If you're still hesitating because you think that only nurse scholars and researchers get their work published, there's more good news! *Dare to Share* is written for nurses who want to write about what they do for nursing magazines, such as *Spectrum* and *Advances in Nursing*; general-practice journals, such as the *American Journal of Nursing* and *Nursing 2008*; specialty-practice journals that run the gamut from infectious disease to hospice care; and books that publish nurses' stories, such as *the HeART of Nursing*,[2] *Ordinary Miracles in Nursing*,[3] and the *Poetry of Nursing*.[4] In Section III, we'll tweak what you've learned about presentations into a step-by-step approach to writing, using a manuscript for a nursing newsletter and a magazine as examples.

Before we begin, let's check in with your three nurse companions. Keri, Betty, and Justin are all interested in "working smart" by turning their presentations into publications. Their free-writes respond to the question, "What presentation are you hoping to turn into a publication in the course of reading this section on writing about what you do?"

Keri writes:

> I'm really glad I didn't try to publish from the get go. Beyond the insights gained in the process of putting my poster presentation together, conference participants raised great questions that gave me loads of ah-hahs. Several of them even encouraged me to publish my findings to reach a broader audience. I came away so jazzed by their responses that I

want to get right on it. I've got a new slant and I'm okay with the writing part. I want to learn more about how to turn my poster into a manuscript.

Betty's entry reads:

I did it! I gave a 15-minute speech at our Nurse's Day dinner entitled, "How Can We Help Each Other Share Our Stories." When the audience gave me a standing ovation, I was in tears. Jon, the hospital newsletter editor, was so impressed by the response that he's asked me to turn my presentation into an article for the next issue. I'm so excited!!! There's only one catch, I have to trim down my speech to a 750-word manuscript. Is there a chapter on pruning in Section III?

Justin wrote:

The capstone course in my BSN program required us to review the literature on a controversial issue in nursing and to present both sides of the argument to our class. My interactive presentation whipped my classmates into such a heated debate on gender preference versus gender bias toward men during educational programs in nursing that my instructor encouraged me to consider submitting an article on this topic. Reading this section is coming at a good time because I want to write a manuscript for the journal *Men in Nursing* while the ideas are still fresh in my mind.

At this point, Keri, Betty, and Justin each have a work-smart strategy in place. It's your turn to free-write your response to the same question they answered in Jot Box 50-1.

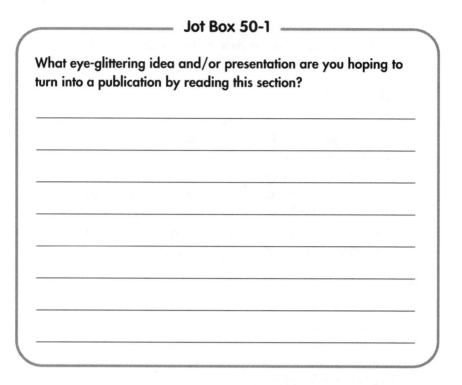

--- **Jot Box 50-1** ---

What eye-glittering idea and/or presentation are you hoping to turn into a publication by reading this section?

Whether the thought of writing about what you do delights or terrifies you, after reading Section III, you'll know how to make it happen.

TIP

Turn the contact high from audience appreciation into the adrenaline rush of seeing your name in print.

References

1. Loomis, A. (2006). *Write from the start: Discover your writing potential through the power of psychological type.* Gainesville, FL: Center for Application of Psychological Type.
2. Wendler, C. (2005). *The heART of nursing: creative expression of art in nursing* (2nd ed.). Indianapolis, IN: Sigma Theta Tau.
3. Winstead-Fry, P., & Labovitz, D. R. (2006). *Ordinary miracles in nursing.* Sudbury, MA: Jones and Bartlett Publishers.
4. Schaefer, J. (Ed.). (2006). *The poetry of nursing: Poems and commentaries of leading nurse-poets.* Kent, OH: Kent State University Press.

I Work Smart

*Hope is a gentle breeze, but fear
is a whipping icy wind.*

Elsie, 8-year-old girl

The other day, an experienced nurse educator told me that she has made 40 presentations and never once published. This is such a common occurrence that I call it the "presenting–publishing barrier." For some nurses, it's a short distance between presenting and publishing, for others the chasm is so wide they can't see to the other side. To find out where you stand, ask yourself the following question: How do my fears about presenting compare with my fears about writing? On the following fearsomeness scale, with 0 being no fear and 10 being yow-zer, attach a number to the following two sharing activities in Jot Box 51-1.

Jot Box 51-1

Fearsomeness Scale

Assign a number to your fear: 0 = No Fear; 10 = Fear Beyond Belief.

Presenting what I do: _____

Writing about what I do: _____

If writing scores higher than presenting, you're not alone. Nurses, as a group, find writing more intimidating than presenting. This should come as no surprise. As a group, we talk far more than we write. Studies have shown that nurses' writing deteriorates between entry into and graduation from nursing programs.[1] After graduation, it used to be that nurses wrote in half-thoughts and fragments—"Vaginal packing in. Doctor out." Now that writing is going the way of dinosaurs with preset textboxes replacing nurses' notes, nurses are writing even less. All of which may explain why nurses' fears about writing trump test-taking when they return to school for advanced degrees.

Even when nurses yearn to share their insights and innovations, their writing efforts can be stifled by offhand remarks or criticisms from someone in the distant past, perhaps a first-grade teacher, or in the present, such as a significant other or a supervisor. Over time, when nurses have no way to respond to these criticisms, the voices of external critics become internalized. These inner critics—think Griselda and Lurch—pepper nurses who suffer from the Impostor Syndrome with self-doubt whenever they dare to write about what they do. So how do you turn a barrier into a bridge? Shift your perspective by working smart and turning your presentations into publications. Ask yourself the perspective-shifting question in Jot Box 51-2.

Jot Box 51-2

What would change in your professional life if you worked smart by turning your presentations into publications?

_____

_____

_____

_____

_____

Like nursing, writing is a practice. With every project and presentation that becomes a publication, you become more of a nurse-author. Make no mistake! Nurse-authors still feel fear whenever they write about what they do; it's just that they don't let their fear paralyze them. They find ways to circumvent inner critiques and criticisms, no matter how clever. As you take on this new identity, you, too, will find yourself throwing around terms like circulation and readership, manuscripts, peer-reviewed journals, and query letters. You'll learn more about each of these terms as they come up in different chapters.

Since you learned how to turn your ideas into a presentation in Section II, you're ready to turn that presentation into a publication. Some of you will welcome this dare to share, others of you will fight it all the way. If you're in the second group, you may surprise yourself. Once you know the steps, you may find yourself enjoying the writing process. No matter which camp you're in, the more you know about yourself as a writer, the easier the writing process will become as you anticipate and negotiate the challenges involved. The more you appreciate what's in it for you to write, not to mention what's in it for your patients, students, or colleagues, the greater your incentive to take the dare to share. We'll start by exploring our inner landscapes as writers.

TIP
Make presenting and publishing companion habits as compatible as cappuccino and dessert.

Reference

1. Diekelmann, N., & Ironside, P. M. (1998). Preserving writing in doctoral education: Exploring the concernful practices of schooling, learning, teaching. *Journal of Advanced Nursing, 28*(6), 1374–1355.

What Makes Writing Easier for You?

52

Make it easy!

Twyla Tharp

Since you first learned to shape your letters with colored crayons, you've spent years writing, first for school and then on the job. Because you write everyday, even if it's only a shopping list, you've probably never thought about what makes writing easier for you. Take a moment to think about it now by completing Jot Box 52-1.

Jot Box 52-1

What's makes writing easier for you?

_____

_____

_____

_____

_____

_____

If you wrote that nothing makes writing easier for you, don't despair. Some of the best nurse-authors I know say there's nothing that makes writing easier. Molly Davison-Price, who peer edited this book and co-authored a chapter in Section 4, is a fine writer who finds the process of writing daunting. She's not good at spelling, and that leaves the door open for her inner critic to give her a hard time. Molly is proof positive that even when there's nothing that makes it easier, you can write about what you do.

If you're going to write about what you do, it's time to learn more about yourself as a writer by exploring how, where, when, and what you write makes the process easier. Compare your answer with the following list of nurses' most common responses during writing workshops to the question "What makes writing easier for me?"

- An idea I know something about
- A conducive setting
- The right equipment
- A block of time

Each of their four responses is explored in more depth here.

An Idea I Know Something About

Chances are the more knowledgeable you are, the greater your incentive to bring attention to a topic by writing about it.

A Conducive Setting

To write, you may need the silence of a library or the noise of a café. Hush or rush, it's important to find a place that's conducive for writing, whether it's as sparse as a monk's cell or filled with things of beauty that appeal to your senses, such as flowers, art, plants, mementoes, or colorful fabrics.

The Right Equipment

As with any sport, the right writing equipment maximizes your comfort as well as your pleasure. Whether it's your PC, a well-gnawed #2 pencil, or a $100.00 Waterman pen, make sure that your writing equipment works for you.

A Block of Time

Blocks of time are nice, but many of us don't have that luxury. It may be more realistic to think in terms of your writing biorhythm. When do you write best? Morning, afternoon, evening? Whenever it's possible to do so, respect your biorhythm by writing during your best time of day. Those of you working shifts or parenting may have to do what poet and writer Tillie Olsen calls "stalking moments of solitude."[1] You wake up earlier or stay up later than everyone else because it's the only quiet time you've got to write.

There's no one right way, there's just your way, to write about what you do. Here's my response to the easier question.

What Makes Writing Easier for Me?

Writing is easiest for me when I'm in my study, music playing in the background to fit my mood, surrounded by my books and files stuffed with articles related to my topic. On a little side table, there's a bouquet of flowers from my garden I look at for inspiration. It's 5:24 AM—my best writing hours are in the early morning. I have my favorite blue cup filled with tea sitting on my desk next to the fat, pink, and golden peach that I picked yesterday. I can hear the birds beginning to twitter and sing as the sky brightens over the water.

Until I answered this question for myself, I never realized what a sensuous experience writing is for me. It's a combination of quiet space, my computer, my favorite food and drink, treasured objects, and familiar sounds that make writing pleasurable. Arrange your writing environment so that it entices you to write. Don't forget to include the sights, sounds, smells, tastes, and feels that make writing easier as you complete Jot Box 52-2.

Jot Box 52-2

Knowing what I know now, I commit to making writing easier for myself by . . .

_____

_____

_____

_____

_____

_____

What makes writing easier is as unique as each writer. So discover your preferences and honor them.

TIP

Make writing easier by creating an environment that invites you to write.

References

1. Olsen, T. (1989). *Silences.* New York: Bantam Doubleday Dell.

What Makes Writing Difficult for You?

53

> *It costs me everything to write, which is really why it's poignant, if not ironic, when critics say, well Maya Angelou has a new book and, of course, it's very good but then she's a natural writer. A natural writer is like a natural heart surgeon.*

Maya Angelou

If writing is difficult for the likes of poet and author Maya Angelou, lighten up on yourself. Everyone's got at least one impediment to writing, so get specific about yours as you answer the question in Jot Box 53-1

Compare what you wrote with the eight challenges that top nurses' lists. Check out the recommended accommodation for the challenge(s) you identified.

The "Where to Start" Challenge—Free-write Accommodation

When getting started is your biggest challenge, beginning a free-write with the phrase "I have no idea where to begin" is like calling on a writing muse who's waiting for you to ask for inspiration. Before the minute is up, you'll find your pen flowing with ideas you never even knew you had. Voila, you've made a start!

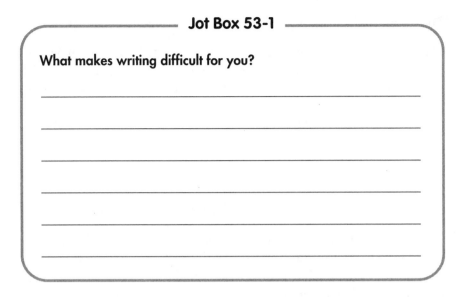

Jot Box 53-1

What makes writing difficult for you?

The "Right Place" Challenge—Artist Date Assignment

When finding the right place to write is your challenge, give yourself artist's dates to try on different settings. You may surprise yourself. Just when you thought the only place you could write is in the hush of a library, you'll find that you're more productive writing at your favorite café warmed by the aroma of coffee and the din of voices. Or that you have different "right places" depending on where you are in the writing process. It may work best to compose on your computer listening to country western music and to revise hard copy versions at a corner table of your favorite restaurant over a late lunch.

The "Time" Challenge—The Chunk-It-Out Accommodation

Nurses are busy people both on and off the job. Don't wait for that week off or you'll never write. Set aside 15 minutes a day to write. Chunk your writing project into 15-minute segments so manuscripts get completed a chunk at a time.

The "Priority" Challenge—The Password Accommodation

When you don't make writing a priority, it goes the way of unscheduled exercise. To protect her writing time, one of my colleague–friends schedules "Writing Appointments" into her date book and arranges her life around these appointments. When you hear yourself saying, "I'd love to meet you for lunch but I have an appointment this afternoon," you'll know you've gotten the "appointment" password down pat and your priorities straight.

The "Impostor" Challenge—The Sweetheart Accommodation

When the Griselda's and Lurch's of inner critics descend upon you, it's time to call in your impostor buster. In this section, you'll meet and find a name for your inner sweetheart—a confident voice to counter even the most wet-blanket messages about writing about what you do.

The "Know How" Challenge—The Strategy and Skill Accommodation

Most nurses don't know how to turn "school papers" into formats acceptable for publication because they were never taught to do so. After reading the *Strategies and Skills* chapters in this section, you'll know how to translate your ideas into publishable products.

The "Voice" Challenge—The *Dare to Share* Notebook Accommodation

Expressing your ideas and opinions in writing takes practice. Expand your entries in your *Dare to Share* notebook to include personal reflections as well as responses to everyday situations. Writing in private can give you the confidence to go public with your writing.

The "Perfectionism" Challenge—The Shitty First Draft

What Accommodation Am I Making to Meet My Biggest Challenge?

Greatest Challenge: The Impostor Challenge

Accommodation: The Sweetheart Accommodation. Whenever I hear Lurch coming after me in his latest disguise designed to derail me from finishing *Dare to Share*, I'm going to call in my Sweetheart (you'll meet her in Chapter 55) to convince Lurch to cease and desist with his attacks.

Accommodation

Jot Box 53-2

What accommodation are you making to meet your biggest challenge?

Greatest Challenge: _____

Accommodation: _____

_____

_____

Allow yourself the creative writer's luxury of the "shitty first draft" (SFD). When you send your SFD to your peer editors, you're that much closer to overcoming the perfectionism challenge.

TIP

Write On! Make accommodations for your writing challenges.

What Are the Benefits of Writing About What You Do?

54

Let me show you how this challenge-accommodation pairing works using my own greatest challenge as an example.

Now it's your turn to identify the accommodation you're going to make to meet your greatest challenge, using Jot Box 53-2.

You're learning a lesson that nurse-authors know well. When writing about what you do, challenges are not an "if," but a "when." So when a challenge comes into view, you'll know how to meet it with an accommodation.

> *Tell me, what is it you plan to do*
> *with your one wild and precious life?*
>
> Mary Oliver

Perhaps you've been so preoccupied with what makes writing difficult that you've never considered what's in it for you. Would it reframe the way you think about writing to consider the benefits and advantages? To see, free-write your response to the question in Jot Box 54-1.

Did you write about the benefits for you, for others, or for a combination of the two? When asked, nurses often speak first about how others benefit from their writing.

Even though it may be more politic in our caring profession to speak about the benefits for others, nurse authors do reap benefits from writing about what they do.

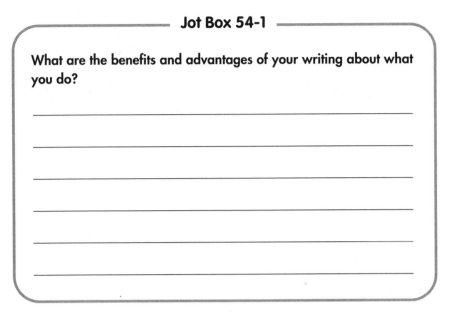

Jot Box 54-1

What are the benefits and advantages of your writing about what you do?

See how your answers compare with the three benefits and advantages nurses identify in writing workshops:

1. Visibility—Spread the word.
2. Credibility—Advance careers and expand professional opportunities.
3. Generativity—Help others by sharing what you've learned.

Each of these benefits are discussed here.

Visibility

Writing about what you do increases the chance that your message will reach the people who need to be reached. You can present to a hundred or even a thousand people, whereas the circulation (the number of subscribers, also referred to as the *readership*) for professional journals can be in the tens of thousands. Unlike presentations that require the time, hassle, and expense of travel, writing allows you to share your ideas with national and international audiences without leaving home.

Credibility

Writing about what you do not only validates the worth of your ideas, it expands professional opportunities and boosts career advancement. Academic nurses are promoted and tenured on the basis of publications and grant proposals; clinicians and nursing leaders practicing in medical centers, such as the one at the University of Southern Maine, apply for sabbatical leaves to study practice-related issues;[1] and nurse entrepreneurs write articles and books to lend authority to the services they offer.

Generativity

Writing is a way to give back to those who have mentored you and to

TIP
Once you see what's in it for you and others, you'll want to write about what you do.

leave a legacy for those coming behind. Readers' calls and e-mails confirm that writing about what you do makes a difference in their lives.

Whether your writing comes from a desire for visibility, credibility, or generativity, as members of the most trusted profession, nurse-authors have tremendous power to influence. We can give a face to a problem, voice the concerns of underserved or disenfranchised groups, and inspire visions of the possible as well as offer practical solutions. Beyond all else, it may be what's in it for your readers, even more than what's in it for you, that keeps you persevering even when the words don't come easily.

References

1. Keefe, S. (2005, June 6). Time for You. *ADVANCE for Nurses New England.* p. 11.

How to Get to Know Your Sweetheart

Let me listen to me and not to them.

Gertrude Stein

In the midst of practicing a new sequences of steps, we all clapped when a woman who'd come to our dance class for about a year shouted, "The voice in my head that used to tell me that I'll never learn these steps is gone!" We knew exactly what she meant. It's that ah-hah moment when you realize that your impostor has left the building. The next time Sue Preneta, our dance teacher, introduced a new routine, this woman's inner critic returned. The difference is that she now knows that she can learn a set of new steps just as she's learned all the others.

How will you know when you've bested your inner critic? My art teacher, Brendan Loughlin, put it well when he said, "I no longer think that I can't do something in a painting, I ask how can I do that." When you turn "I can't" into "How can I?" you'll know that you're no longer in the grip of your imposter. You develop, in other words, an inner voice to counter your inner critic's doubts, fears, and judgments. Natalie Goldberg, who writes inspirational books for creative writers, calls this voice your "sweetheart."[1] Writing to your inner sweetheart diminishes the tendency to "...believe criticism more than positive feedback" (p. 56).[1] To show you what an inner sweetheart sounds like, here's a letter I wrote to mine.

231

Letter

Kathy: Dearest Sweetheart, I find myself needing you more than ever as I start to work on the final drafts of this book. The closer *Dare to Share* gets to being finished, the more Lurch is wearing me down with complaints and criticisms. What I'm writing is no good. Who would want to read this? What am I thinking trying to write a book anyway? If I'm not careful, I'll believe him. Every day it gets harder to make myself go to my study. My biggest fear is that I'll just give up and this book will never get published. Can you help me?

Sweetheart: If you let me, I can help.

Kathy: How?

Sweetheart: When you hear Lurch begin to criticize, it's time to switch your attention to me. I'll remind you of the time when you were a new grad working on a psychiatric unit and your supervisor looked up from reading a nurse's note you'd written and said, "This is just like a novel, I can't put it down. You're a wonderful writer." Or all the times when nurse reviewers who didn't even agree with what you wrote started their critiques with the words, "This is well-written." Or, when Marilyn Oermann called out of the blue to ask you to co-edit *The Annual Review of Nursing Education* because she enjoys your writing style and shares your articles with her students.

Kathy: Just having you remind me of those things does take the sting out of my impostor's critical questions. Although I can still hear him whispering, "Yeah, that was then and this is now. You've never tried to write a book before."

Sweetheart: If you asked, I'd tell you that a book is just like a collection of articles. Instead of articles, they're chapters. So this really isn't the first time you've written a book, it's just the first time you've strung a bunch of articles into a book.

Kathy: So for each criticism, you come back with a positive, is that how this works?

Sweetheart: Yeah, pretty much. All you have to do is ask for help. Then I'll wear Lurch down with positives to counter his negatives. And, in doing so, I remind you to hold onto the value of what you are doing. That's when Lurch loses his power to bring you down.

Having that dialogue with my sweetheart just now helped me to recover my inner balance. It's time to give your sweetheart a voice (see Jot Box 55-1). As you can see, mine was not so much a letter as a conversation. Allow your communication to take whatever form fits you and your sweetheart best. If this letter doesn't come easily at first, keep your pen moving and you'll be amazed at how inventive your sweetheart is in countering even the most sour-voiced inner critic.

Jot Box 55-1

Dear Sweetheart:

_____

_____

_____

_____

_____

_____

How do you feel having written a letter to your sweetheart? Once you establish contact, you can write your sweetheart whenever you're feeling shaky or impostorish, 24/7. It's very good timing, because if you thought your inner critic was raging when you broached the idea of presenting, see what happens when you want to write about what you do. This is why it's as important to name your sweetheart as it was to name your inner critic (see Jot Box 55-2). I call mine Kate because she's as feisty and clear-sighted and good at defending me as Katharine Hepburn, one of my idols, was at defending herself. As you can see from my sweetheart letter, Kate's more than a match for Lurch, my grouchy inner critic. In the event that you have trouble coming up with a name for your inner ally, write him or her a note to ask what he or she would prefer being called.

Jot Box 55-2

Your inner sweetheart is named. . .

_____

Welcome your inner sweetheart to your support circle and write him or her often and always when your inner critic is causing mischief.

TIP
Writing to your Sweetheart self is not only free, it's freeing.

Reference

1. Goldberg, N. (1990). *Wild mind: living the writer's life.* New York: Bantam New Age Books.

How Would You Describe Your Writing Style?

56

> *. . . we ought not grope for our one true voice so much as we should pay attention to the manifold voices that resound across the landscape. One could argue that the inability or unwillingness to evolve in such a fashion has led more than a few of our strongest writers to silence . . .*

Andrew Furman

Jan, a photographer and freelance writer, wanted a doctoral degree to give her the credibility she needed to author books. After four years of writing academic papers, not to mention a dissertation, Jan thought she'd drop off her academic writing style along with her graduation robe. She was shocked to find that somewhere along the way she'd lost her breezy, women's magazine style. It would take her several years to recover her informal writing style, but this time it wasn't really her old style. This new writing style was somewhere in between casual and academ-ese.

Just as you have a presenting style, you also have a writing style. Take Jan, for instance. If we gave Jan's various author-voices names, her freelance voice was that of a Casual Observer; her doctoral student voice that of a Formal Academic; and her author-voice after graduation settled into that of an Informed Conversationalist. Laid along a continuum, Jan's three writing styles as she morphed from journalist to book author would look like this:

[Jan the Journalist]	[Jan the Published Author]	[Jan the Doctoral Student]
Casual Observer	Informed Conversationalist	Formal Academic
←		→
First person	First person	Third person
Few references	More references	Lots of references
Contractions	Contractions	No contractions

What about you? If you're not sure whether your writing style is more that of a Casual Observer, an Informed Conversationalist, or a Formal Academic, let's start with a reading sample. Which of the following two versions of Diana and Kelley's chapter on poster presentations is more appealing to you?

Version 1

Because posters are a visual medium, white space should organize the sections into a neat and orderly learning tool. Posters can flow in one of two ways, by columns or rows. Although both schemes can work, gravity naturally pulls the eyes from top to bottom, then left to right. When using rows, the viewer usually needs to stop and turn his or her head to read the content of the poster.[2]

After reading this next passage, make a decision about which version is more appealing.

Version 2

We wanted to make a visual impact with our poster. Given that we might or might not be present when our poster was viewed, our poster had to be self-explanatory and concise in relaying outcomes and achievements.[2] In other words, it would need to attract attention and "stand on its own" in terms of the viewer being able to clearly discern content. To keep the poster readable, we used white space to organize the information. From our reading, we learned that posters can flow in one of two ways, by columns or rows. Although both schemes can work, gravity naturally pulls the eyes from top to bottom, then left to right. When using rows, the viewer usually needs to stop and turn his or her head to read the content of the poster.[2] With this in mind, our poster has three columns with three slides in the first two columns and four slides in the third column.

Remember that you're stating your preference here; there is no right or wrong answer. Which version did you enjoy reading more? Version 1 is a third-person account; whereas Version 2 is a first-person approach. The "they" of third person distances the author from the readers; the "I/we" of first person is more up close and personal.

In Jot Box 56-1, check off the type(s) of nursing magazines or journals that you prefer to read.

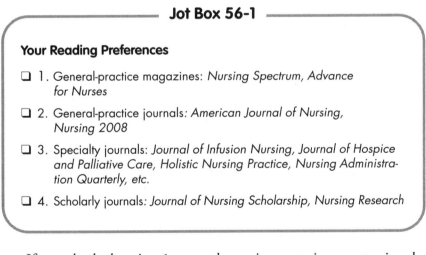

Jot Box 56-1

Your Reading Preferences

❑ 1. General-practice magazines: *Nursing Spectrum, Advance for Nurses*

❑ 2. General-practice journals: *American Journal of Nursing, Nursing 2008*

❑ 3. Specialty journals: *Journal of Infusion Nursing, Journal of Hospice and Palliative Care, Holistic Nursing Practice, Nursing Administration Quarterly,* etc.

❑ 4. Scholarly journals: *Journal of Nursing Scholarship, Nursing Research*

If you checked option 1, general-practice magazines, you enjoy the writing of Casual Observers. Because you read as much to be entertained as to be informed, you prefer articles written in the first person without a lot of quoting from experts. If you chose 3, specialty journals, you appreciate the writing of Informed Conversationalists who engage your interest by writing in the first person and referencing the latest thinking and research on the topic in intriguing ways. If option 4, scholarly journals, was your choice, you enjoy being intellectually stimulated by scholarly articles and books written in the third person that is consistent with the Formal Academic style. These theoretical pieces are grounded in experts' ideas and research findings followed by lengthy reference lists.

Now let's talk about you as a writer. Are you more comfortable writing in the first or third person? As a child in school, you were taught to write like a Formal Academic, referring to yourself as "the author." Indeed, writing in the third person is a standard requirement for school papers, theses, dissertations, and scholarly publications. Even when they prefer to read the writing of Casual Observers or Informed Conversationalists, nurses often find it daunting to shift from writing in the third person to the first person. As one nurse author wrote:

> After so many years of writing in academ-ese, I'm really having trouble writing in the first person. It makes me feel very vulnerable, as if I don't have any clothes on. There are no experts for me to hide behind. When readers know it's me doing the writing, they can hold me accountable for what I say. Whew, now there's a scary thought!

Once you try it, you may find that you enjoy writing in the first person used by Informed Conversationalists or Casual Observers, but it's going to take time and practice before it feels like it's your preferred writing style.

Take a minute to consider the writing style that comes most naturally to you in Jot Box 56-2.

Jot Box 56-2

Your Reading Preferences

❑ a. Casual Observer

❑ b. Informed Conversationalist

❑ c. Formal Academic

There's no question that your preferred writing style is your comfort zone. If you're a scholar/researcher who's always written in the third person or if you've never written for publication before, stretch yourself. Just as you can speak in a high, chipmunk voice or a low sultry voice, use big words or small words, the King's English or slang, over the course of your nursing career, take opportunities to add Informed Conversational or Casual Observer styles to your repertoire of writing styles. Then you'll be able to write about what you do in the style that best fits your topic and your target audience. The more versatile you are in transitioning from one writing style to another, the easier it will be for you to share what you do with a variety of readers.

TIP

To return to your preferred writing style after writing in another style can be as refreshing as sorbet after a spicy dish.

How to Write Yourself into Still-Point

57

Who looks outside, dreams.
Who looks inside, awakens.

Carl Jung

In a section devoted to writing, it's only fitting that you try writing your way into still-point, especially since the types of writing nurses do often constricts our thinking to bullet points. This still-point strategy, like stretching before exercising, is meant to warm up your mental joints and muscles to increase your suppleness and flexibility as a writer. For this free-write, an adaptation of two free-writing approaches—"morning papers"[1] and Proprioceptive Writing[2]—you'll need the following:

- 10 minutes
- A quiet place where you won't be disturbed
- A timer or stopwatch
- A writing implement
- A candle
- Baroque music
- An entry in your *Dare to Share* notebook *or* five sheets of blank, unlined paper

Why was I so specific about Baroque music?

> . . . Baroque music has a calming effect on the body, including lowering blood pressure; that its slower tempo, which have roughly the same number of beats per minute as the human heart, shifts the brain off its everyday beta rhythms to alpha rhythms that are more conducive to creativity and learning (p. 28).[2]

Once you've gathered all you need, place your pen and paper on the writing surface in front of you.

Start the music, light your candle, set the timer for 10 minutes, cup your hands over your eyes, and take three deep breaths with the intention of clearing your mind of distractions. Then allow yourself to write whatever comes to mind, trusting that whatever you write is exactly what needs to be written.

How was that for you? In the beginning, some nurses find it hard to begin, but once they get going they don't want to stop. Lulled by the Baroque music, they write themselves into a receptive place by exploring their:

- Thoughts or feelings related to a situation in their lives
- Ideas for writing projects
- Solutions for a life-related or writing challenge

How do these compare with what you wrote about?

This still-point strategy is one to cultivate when you want your ideas to flow unfettered from mind to paper. Writing yourself into still-point—creating transitional space with Baroque music, setting your intention for your creative task, lighting a candle, cupping hands over eyes, and taking three deep breaths—prepares you to write about what you do. Practice increases proficiency. When you use your *Dare to Share* notebook, you'll free-write your way into some writing ideas as well as record them for future use. Talk about working smart!

TIP

Write yourself into still-point to release the flow of your thoughts and feelings, your memories, and dreams.

References

1. Cameron, J., with Bryan, M. (1992). *The artist's way: a spiritual path to higher creativity.* New York: G.P. Putnam's Sons.
2. Trichter Metcalf, L., & Tobin, S. (2002). *Writing the mind alive: The proprioceptive method for finding your authentic voice.* New York: Ballantine Books.

How to See if Your Idea Has Enough Eye-Glitter for a Publication

58

Don't tell me you can't write. You're a nurse, you can do anything. What you can accomplish in a day would put most other professionals to shame.

Joan Borgatti

Do you have a presentation that you want to turn into a manuscript? Or are you starting with a new idea? It doesn't matter, because wherever you begin, the process of writing about what you do involves the following three small steps: (1) clarify your idea in a free-write; (2) assign your idea an eye-glitter score; and (3) complete a Publication Worksheet.

Step 1: Free-Write

To become a writer, you must begin to "think writing" by asking yourself what happened today that you can write about. For me, my inspiration for a publication came from a presentation. When viewed through a "what's write-up-able about this" lens, you'll find inspiration all around you in your practice, everyday conversations and in the presentations that you've given. See my example on the following page, then try it yourself in Jot Box 58-1.

What Happened to Me Today that I Could Write About?

When I awoke this morning, after presenting to the school nurses' group last night, I wanted to redo my presentation. How could I share the 10 steps they'd taught me for dealing with joy-stealing? All of a sudden, I flashed on Lisa Nowak's showing me a copy of this group's newsletter. Right then and there I decided to email her to ask about publishing a newsletter article related to the 10 steps.

Jot Box 58-1

What happened to you today that you could write about?

_____

_____

_____

_____

_____

_____

_____

What do you notice as you reread your free-write? Did a presentation spawn a new idea for a publication? Or did something happen to you that's just begging to be written? Were you unsure that anything of note happened until an idea pulsating with possibility appeared in your free-write? If your free-write didn't spark any ideas, not to worry. Make a habit of asking yourself this free-write question. With practice, your powers of finding writing opportunities all around you will increase along with your ability to translate everyday events into inspirational material for your writing projects.

When you've got an idea or maybe even a couple of ideas, you're ready to move onto the next step.

Step 2: Plot Your Idea's Eye-Glitter Score

Remember this fun step in selecting an idea for a presentation? As you can see, I use the same procedure to find out whether my idea has the eye-glitter score to keep me inspired during the writing process.

Least Glitter				Moderate Glitter				Most Glitter		
0	1	2	3	4	5	6	7	8	9	10

The Eye-Glitter Scale

I'm thrilled to report that my "joy-stealer is me" idea is a 10+, what's yours?

Least Glitter				Moderate Glitter				Most Glitter		
0	1	2	3	4	5	6	7	8	9	10

The Eye-Glitter Scale

Make sure that your idea has a high enough eye-glitter score to keep you interested enough to turn it into a publishable product.

Step 3: Complete A Publication Worksheet

Once you've isolated an idea with enough eye-glitter for your writing project, it's time to complete a Publication Worksheet. Although most of the items are the same as those on the Presentation Worksheet, it's obvious from the cross-outs and substitutions on the following blank Publication Worksheet that there's been a few changes.

Publication Worksheet

Idea: _____

_____

Topic: _____

Focus: _____

Purpose: _____

~~Audience~~ **Readers:** _____

~~Venue~~ **Vehicle:** _____

Desired ~~Audience~~ Reader Response: _____

Slant (Title): _____

One-sentence description: This article will _____

Three items have changed—readers, vehicle, and desired reader responses. These will be discussed in the following three chapters so you'll know all you need to know to complete your Publication Worksheet.

TIP

Like a miner sifting for gold, sift through your experiences for eye-glittering ideas.

How Choosing Your Readership Decides Your Vehicle

59

Write for your readers.

Suzanne Hall Johnson

As you can see from his e-mail message below, Mike knew he wanted to write his first article for the lay public before he knew what he wanted to write about:

> Well, it took me five long years to do it, but I finally graduated from the MSN program . . .When I took your course in 2001, I told you it was my 'dream' to write for the popular press, because I felt it was a nurse's responsibility to educate people outside of nursing. What better way to reach an audience than in a publication that they actually read!
>
> Well, I have reached this goal. I submitted an article to *Modern Drummer Magazine*, titled "Back Safety: Every Drummer's Responsibility," and it is scheduled for publication in the coming months. I have you, as well as my other instructors over the past five years, to thank for believing that it was possible for a nurse to get published in media intended for other professions.
>
> Mike Bafuma, MSN, RN (My goodness, it feels nice to write that!)

There are two types of readers you can write for: the lay public and professional colleagues. The readership for my project was a group of professionals. Check off the readers whom you want to reach with your writing project in Jot Box 59-1.

Jot Box 59-1

Readership for your project:
❏ a. Lay public
❏ b. Professional

Your readership determines your *vehicle*—where you want to publish your piece. If, like Mike, you want to write for the lay public, you'll publish in a popular press vehicle. If, like me, you want to write for a professional audience, you'll search for a professional vehicle. Popular press vehicles, like *Modern Drummer's World*, target a segment of readers in the general public and include online blogs or e-zines, newspapers, magazines, e-books, and books. Professional press vehicles address specialized audiences. These include newsletters, magazines, and journals that are either online or off-line, monographs, e-books, and books. In the case of books for lay or professional audiences, nurse-authors may self-publish or enlist the services of a publishing company, such as Jones and Bartlett Publishers. So what type of vehicle are you seeking for your manuscript?

Jot Box 59-2

Your type of vehicle:
❏ a. Popular press
❏ b. Professional vehicle

Although there is increasing interest among nurses in publishing in popular vehicles, the reality is that most nurses write for professional colleagues in nursing periodicals. *Periodicals* are vehicles published at specific time intervals (e.g., weekly, bi-weekly, monthly, bi-monthly, etc.) According to the Cornell University Library, there are four types of periodical literature: scholarly, substantive news/general interest, popular, and sensational.[1] Unless you know something I don't, there's no sensational, *National Enquirer*–type publications in nursing. Adapting this schema for our purposes, nursing periodicals will be divided into three categories depending on the readership: general interest, substantive news, and scholarly.

General Interest	Substantive News	Scholarly
Generalists	Specialty Practitioners	Scholars/Researchers

Type of Professional Periodical and Readership Continuum

If you want to write for a professional audience, determine which professional colleagues you want to write for using Jot Box 59-3. My writing project targets the specialty practice of nurse educators.

Jot Box 59-3

Your writing project targets this professional group:
❑ Generalists
❑ Specialty practitioners
❑ Scholars/researchers

Having decided what group you want to write for, what writing style would best fit them? You'll narrow your choices for professional vehicles by deciding this up front, because different professional vehicles require different writing styles. In general, articles in scholarly nursing periodicals discuss theoretical concepts or summarize research studies using a formal-academic style and are written in the third person with lengthy reference lists. There are some exceptions, as in the case of the scholarly journal *Advances in Nursing Science (ANS)*, edited by Dr. Peggy Chinn, in which writing in an informed conversational writing style is acceptable. Substantive news/general interest periodicals often describe applications to practice and are written in the first person in an informed conversational style with fewer references than scholarly vehicles.

General Interest (Generalists)	Substantive News (Specialty Practitioners)	Scholarly (Scholars/Researchers)
Casual Observer	Informed Conversational	Formal Academic

Type of Professional Periodical and Readership Continuum

With this in mind, what writing style do you want to use to write to your target audience of readers (Jot Box 59-4)?

Jot Box 59-4

You want to write to your readers using this writing style:
❑ Casual Observer
❑ Informed Conversational
❑ Formal Academic

Keeping your readership and writing style preference in mind, let's take a moment to discuss the reference books that can guide your project. If, like Mike, you want to publish in the popular press, there are two resources you'll want to own. *From Silence to Voice: What Nurses Know and Must Communicate to the Public*,[2] is a complete guide to breaking into the popular press. If, like best-selling author Sue Monk Kidd, you're a nurse wanting to learn more about creative writing, the most highly regarded periodical is *Poets & Writers: From Inspiration to Publication*. In addition to interviews with authors and all sorts of relevant information, it lists conferences that introduce creative writers to the craft as well as the business of getting manuscripts accepted for publication. If you're serious about learning the craft of writing, consider subscribing to *The Writer's Chronicle: A Publication of the Association of*

Writers and Writing Programs. The *Writer's Market,* a yearly publication, offers helpful information about getting manuscripts published, from choosing agents to vehicles. *Dare to Share* is the book to read when you want to write for professional vehicles in the general information and substantive news category. If you're more interested in writing in research or scholarly publications, particularly if you're a new faculty member, then you'd do well to purchase *Scholarly and Career Development: Strategies for Success*[4] which is billed as a scholarship manual for NP faculty. Or if you want to learn more about the writing process and ethical and legal issues, then Marilyn Oermann's *Writing for Publication in Nursing* is for you.[3]

Now you can appreciate Suzanne Hall Johnson's suggestion to write for your readers, because that decision determines your writing style and narrows the options for potential vehicles.

TIP
Decide for whom you want to write and decisions about writing style and vehicle will follow.

References

1. *Cornell University Library. (2007).* Distinguishing scholarly journals from other periodicals. *Retrieved August 20, 2007, from http://www.library.cornell.edu/olinuris/ref/research/skill20.html*
2. Buresh, B., & Gordon, S. (2000). *From silence to voice: What nurses know and must communicate to the public.* Ottawa, Ontario: Canadian Nurses Association.
3. Oermann, M. H. (2002). *Writing for publication in nursing.* Philadelphia: Lippincott, Williams & Wilkins.
4. National Organization of Nurse Practitioner Faculties. (2005). *Scholarship and career development: Strategies for success.* Washington, DC: Author.

How to Select Potential Professional Vehicles

60

Identify possible journals first, select the top one on that list, and write the manuscript FOR the journal.

Marilyn H. Oermann

With more than 540 nursing and allied health periodicals to choose from,[1] how do you find the "best home" for your work? Instead of thinking of yourself as a reader, start thinking of yourself as a nurse-author and detective combined, and you're halfway there. Now that you've got your Sherlock Holmes hat on, the next step is identifying the general category of professional periodical that best fits your focused topic and readers:

1. General practice
2. Specialty practice
3. Administrative
4. Educational
5. Professional development
6. Scholarly/research

The category of periodical that best fits my topic is educational. Write down your response to the question in Jot Box 60-1.

Jot Box 60-1

What category of periodical best fits your topic/readers?

_____

With this decided, you're ready to narrow your possibilities even more. In the last chapter, you learned that there are three categories of nursing periodicals: general interest for generalists, substantive news for nurses in various nursing specialties, and scholarly for scholars and researchers. Table 60-1 offers an example of each vehicle.

TABLE 60-1   Type of Nursing Periodical, Readership, Format, and Examples

Type	Readership	Format	Example
General interest	Generalists	E-zine	*Nurse.com e-zine*
		Magazine	*Advance for Nurses*
		Journal	*Nursing 2008*
Substantive news	Clinicians, educators, and scholars	Magazine	*Reflections on Nursing Leadership (RNL)*
	Educators	Specialty Journal	*Nursing Education Perspectives*
	Administrators	Specialty Journal	*Journal of Nursing Administration*
	Clinicians in specialty practice	Specialty Journal	*Journal of Operating Room Nursing*
	Continuing education and staff development educators	Specialty Journal	*Journal of Continuing Education*
Scholarly	Scholar/Researcher	Journal	*Journal of Nursing Scholarship*

Notice how I used the information in this table as a guide to complete the items in the box on the following page.

My Writing Project

Type of nursing periodical: Substantive news

Readership: Educators

Format(s): Magazine or journal

Using Table 60-1 as a guide, complete the questions in Jot Box 60-2.

Jot Box 60-2

Your Writing Project

Type of nursing periodical: _____

Readership: _____

Format(s): _____

Now that you've identified the type of periodical that best fits your topic and readers, you're ready to develop a list of periodicals. There are three ways to do this:

1. *Review* the periodicals that you read.
2. *Ask* nurse-authors who write for your readership for suggestions.
3. *Conduct* your own search.

When I reviewed the magazines and journals that I read on a regular basis, three possible vehicles came to mind for the "joy-stealer" project (see the following page).

In this case, I felt confident enough about these three choices that I didn't feel the need to expand on my search or ask colleagues for suggestions.

Vehicles for Joy-Stealing Manuscript

Reflections on Nursing Leadership—Online professional magazine
Nurse Educator—Professional journal
Nursing Education Perspectives—Professional journal (also available online)

Now it's your turn. If you've never written before, I'd suggest that you complete these three steps in whatever sequence fits you and your project. Should your search for vehicles require it, why not make the library a destination for one of your artist's dates? With online magazines and journals, save the gas and complete your article-by-article search for vehicles on your home PC. Whether at the library or online, you're searching for vehicles whose mission and readership best fit your topic and target audience. It's easy when the target readership is contained in the title of the periodical, as in the case of the following three journals for academic nurses: *Nurse Educator, Nursing Education Perspectives,* and *Journal of Nursing Education.* Your detective skills come in very handy when you can't tell the readership by reading the title of the periodical. For example, Sigma Theta Tau International Honor Society publishes an online nursing magazine quarterly called *Reflections on Nursing Leadership (RNL).* The mission of *RNL* is "...to communicate, through informative articles, biographic profiles and personal narratives the vitally important contributions that nurses make toward improving world health." Although you can't tell from this description, a review of the chapters in any issue would tell you that the *RNL* readership is largely academic nurses, which is my target audience. That's why it's important to look beyond titles to thumb through volumes while reviewing articles with an eye to readership as well as topics.

Once you've identified several possible vehicles, review a year's worth of volumes for topics published, writing style, and the formatting of articles. From each vehicle, make a copy of an article with a topic similar to yours written in a person/writing style compatible with yours. Then, should you choose this periodical as your vehicle, you'll have the format to follow for outlining your own manuscript. As you begin your investigation, whether in person or virtual, consider the following three "work smart" principles for locating potential vehicles:

1. **Start small, enjoy success, move on**. When possible, write your first piece for a vehicle that fits your preferred writing style, whether it's a letter to the editor of your hospital newsletter or an article for *Nursing Spectrum*. Once you experience the high of seeing your name in print, stretching your writing style to author manuscripts for other types of vehicles will follow.

2. **Mix and match**. When the topic lends itself, write an article for two different audiences: One for a lay audience in the popular press and one for a professional audience in a nursing vehicle. Then you're not only spreading the word about your topic, you're spreading the word about nurses and nursing!

3. **Don't put all your eggs in one vehicle**. The goal of this investigation is to find several vehicles—I like to find three potential vehicles per writing project—that look promising. When you line up several potential vehicles, should the editor of your first choice reject your manuscript, you have other options.

Now that you know all you need to know to begin your search—have fun! Once you compile a list with several possibilities, you're ready to complete Jot Box 60-3.

Jot Box 60-3

Three Potential Vehicles:

1. _____

2. _____

3. _____

Lavish time and energy on searching for the perfect vehicle. Then when your article is published, you'll have the satisfaction of knowing your message is reaching your target readership.

> **TIP**
> Make an adventure out of searching for a vehicle that's a perfect fit for your readers.

References

1. *Cornell University Library. (2007).* Distinguishing scholarly journals from other periodicals. *Retrieved August 20, 2007, from http://www.library.cornell. edu/olinuris/ref/research/skill20.html*

How to Elicit Your Desired Reader Response

Have a target journal and focus on those readers when you write. Write for the reader. Ask yourself what they would want to know about your topic.

Suzanne Hall Johnson

As a presenter, you're face-to-face with your audience participants. You can tell how a presentation is going from the expressions on their faces, the feeling in the room, and their questions and comments. For authors, this feedback loop is missing. Writing is a one-way conversation with readers whom you cannot see and who rarely get or take the opportunity to share their responses with you. That's why, when this reader reached out to me, I was so excited I had to write to Jim Mattson, editor of *Reflections on Nursing Leadership (RNL)*, to tell him about it:[1]

> I got a call last night from an 80-year-old retired nurse who lives on a 97-acre farm in Indiana. She wanted me to know that my joy-stealing article [Second Qtr. 2006] touched her and if I need any more stories, she's got plenty. She can't wait to read the second article!

Talk about a desired reader response; having a reader call me was a first in my career as a nurse-author. Our phone conversation, along with a number of impassioned e-mail messages from other readers, confirmed that my purpose for writing this article—to "awaken, arouse, and activate"—was more than fulfilled.

Whether it's conscious or not, your purpose for writing is to elicit a response in your readers. To see how reader response connects with the purpose for writing a piece, let's look at my current writing project.

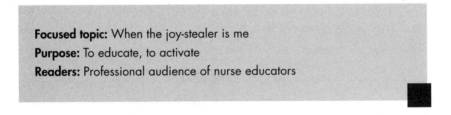

Focused topic: When the joy-stealer is me
Purpose: To educate, to activate
Readers: Professional audience of nurse educators

Table 61-1 matches the desired reader response and purpose.

TABLE 61-1 Purpose and Desired Reader Response

Purpose	Desired Reader Response
1. Educate	Learn something
2. Awaken, arouse, and activate	Act on a problem
3. Inspire	Manifest a vision of the possible
4. Advertise	Buy product
5. Gain professional recognition	Give accolades that merit awards, certifications, promotion, tenure, pay raises
6. Obtain personal satisfaction	Report that life has been changed by reading this publication

Since my purpose was to education and activate, see how I answered the following question.

My Desired Reader Response is that they are moved to stop joy-stealing game playing based on what they've learned.

My purpose for changing the item "audience response" on the Presentation Worksheet to "reader response" on the Publication Worksheet is to elicit a response in you, dear reader. I want to move you to establish a personal connection with *your* readers. Instead of focusing on what you want to say, ask what it is your readers want to know. If you're not sure, ask colleagues who fit the description of your readers what they would want to know. Write every manuscript as if it were a letter to your readers. Start now by deciding which type of reader response you are seeking based on your purpose for writing this manuscript in the first place (use Jot Box 61-1).

Jot Box 61-1

Focused topic: _____

Purpose: _____

Readers: _____

Your Desired Reader Response is _____

_____

_____

When you consider the type of response you're seeking from readers, you'll write *to them*, as well as for them. Doing so not only enlivens your writing, it guides decisions about what to include, and perhaps even more important, what to delete.

TIP

When your readers respond as you hoped they would, yours is a message that resonates.

References

1. Heinrich, K. T. (2006, Third Quarter). Letter to Editor. *Reflections on Nursing Leadership*. Available at www.nursingsociety.org

How Presentation Worksheets Become Publication Worksheets

62

> *Adventures don't begin until you get into the forest. That first step is an act of faith.*

Mickey Hart

When you work smart by translating a Presentation Worksheet into a Publication Worksheet, the very act of presenting and interacting with audience-participants results in the items on the Publication Worksheet becoming more specific. To show you how these differences can look, I break down the differences between my Presentation and Publication Worksheets item by item below.

Item	Presentation Worksheet	Publication Worksheet
Idea	Joy stealing	Joy-stealing games
Topic	Joy-stealing games	What school nurses can do to stop the game-playing
Focus	What school nurses need to know about joy-stealing games	Ten steps to stop the joy-stealing

As you can see, the topic on the Presentation Worksheet becomes the Idea on the Publication Worksheet, which makes for a more detailed topic and focus.

This trend continues with the purpose for the publication being more exact than that of the presentation, as shown here.

Item	Presentation Worksheet	Publication Worksheet
Purpose	To educate and awaken school nurses to joy-stealing games and introduce strategies for establishing zestful relationships with students, teachers, administrators, and parents.	To give back to school nurse group by sharing lessons they taught me about 10 steps in stopping joy-stealing.

Notice that the purposes of educating and awakening become "give back to" in the Publication Worksheet.

I compare and contrast the rest of the items on each worksheet below.

Item	Presentation Worksheet	Publication Worksheet
Audience/ Readership	110 school nurses	Association of School Nurses of CT
Venue/Vehicle	Restaurant dining room	*The Pulse of ASNC Newsletter*
Desired Audience/ Reader Response	To foster zestful school environments with zero-tolerance for such games	To inform and move school nurses to use the strategies to halt the joy-stealing
Slant (Title)	Joy Stealing: What School Nurses Can Do to Stop The Mean Games	What CT School Nurses Taught Me About Stopping Joy-stealing

Instead of the 110 audience-participants who attended this dinner presentation, the readership on the Publication Worksheet expands to include the entire membership who receives the association's newsletter. The trend toward specificity continues with desired reader response focusing on 10 strategies rather than more global zero-tolerance. So, too, the slant shifts from the more general "what school nurses can do" to the more delineated "what CT nurses taught me." It stands to reason that association newsletter readers would be interested in reading what their colleagues have to say about joy-stealing.

See how the one-sentence description on the Presentation Worksheet speaks to what *might* happen, whereas the Publication Worksheet description turns what *did* happen in the presentation into the central idea for a manuscript.

Item	Presentation Worksheet	Publication Worksheet
One-Sentence Description	Designed to stimulate spirited dialogue, this interactive session engages participants in sharing stories about situations that stole their joy and strategizing new ways of responding that foster zestful academic environments.	This newsletter article describes what I learned from school nurses about 10 steps for stopping the joy-stealing games.

Now that you've seen the differences between my two worksheets, it's time for you to complete your own Publication Worksheet on the following page.

Publication Worksheet		
Item	Presentation Worksheet	Publication Worksheet
Idea	_____	_____
Topic	_____	_____
Focus	_____	_____
Audience/Readership	_____	_____
Venue/Vehicle	_____	_____
Desired Audience/ Reader Response	_____	_____
Slant/Title	_____	_____
One-Sentence Description	_____	_____

If you have not already done so, copy the information from your Presentation and/or Publication Worksheets into the Appendices (see Appendix A and Appendix C). Then whenever you need to refer to either of both of them, you'll know exactly where to find your completed worksheets.

TIP

When you work smart, Publication Worksheet items will be more specific than your Presentation Worksheet items.

How to Write Queries That Sell Editors on Your Idea

63

Make your query appeal to that particular editor's readership. Point out in your query how his/her readership can benefit from the article and how it fits a need in the magazine/newspaper.

Joan Borgatti

To query or not to query? Now that you've selected the vehicle(s) that best fits your message and your audience, you've got a choice to make. While this is a good time to query editors about their interest in reviewing your manuscript, it's an optional step that many nurse-authors skip. I include this step in my workshops for a number of reasons. In addition to narrowing your options, a well-written query can become the introduction to your manuscript, help you make the transition from worksheets to the actual writing process, and give you a gentle introduction into peer editing.

For authors, sending queries *is* working smart. When editors accept queries, and not all of them do, it makes sense to translate the one-sentence description from your Publication Worksheet into a query tailored to a specific audience. Given the speed of electronic communications, most editors respond to queries within 24 to 72 hours. This makes it possible, before you even review the literature or make an outline, to know which editor(s) and which vehicle(s) are interested in your manuscript. Beyond being buoyed by the knowledge that a specific editor is interested, your manuscript can be written in a vehicle-ready format.

This chapter shares a brief and a longer, more formal format for queries that illustrate the essential components before you outline your own. Because I'd already published two articles on joy-stealing in *Reflections on Nursing Education* (*RNL*) last summer, I worked smart by querying *RNL* editor, Jim Mattson about his interest in my latest manuscript idea:

Query

Kathleen T. Heinrich wrote:

Re: *What to Do When the Joy-Stealer Is Me?*

Dear Jim:

Happy New Year! RNL readers' email response to the second joy-stealing article was so vigorous, I hope you'll consider publishing a third article in the series with the working title "What to Do When the Joy-Stealer Is Me?"

This article is written to help readers explore how they steal joy from students, colleagues and administrators; to deepen their compassion for joy-stealers; and to initiate dialogues about joy-stealing in faculty meetings, classrooms and clinical settings.

Thanks as always for your kind consideration!!

Kathy

Kathleen T. Heinrich RN, PhD
Principal
K T H Consulting
Business Address
Business Phone Number
Web Site Address

Let's examine this query from two perspectives: form and function. *Form* relates to the six components that make queries complete:

1. Working title of manuscript as heading
2. Greeting with the name of editor: "Dear . . ."
3. One-sentence description (from Publication Worksheet)

4. Appeal for readership
5. Formal closing
6. Contact information

It's good form, for example, to begin your queries with a greeting/ salutation of "Dear" and the name of the editor. Had I not worked with Jim before, I would have addressed him in the greeting/salutation as "Mr. Mattson." The six components for complete queries are labeled on my query below.

Query

Kathleen T. Heinrich wrote:
Re: *What to Do When the Joy-Stealer Is Me?* ——— **Working title**

Dear Jim:—**Greeting/salutation**

Highlight appeal for readership

Happy New Year! RNL readers' email response to the second joy-stealing article was so vigorous, I hope you'll consider publishing a third article in the series with the working title "What to Do When the Joy-Stealer Is Me?"

One-sentence description

This article is written to help readers explore how they steal joy from students, colleagues and administrators; to deepen their compassion for joy-stealers; and to initiate dialogues about joy-stealing in faculty meetings, classrooms and clinical settings.

Formal sign-off

Thanks as always for your kind consideration!!
Kathy

Kathleen T. Heinrich RN, PhD
Principal
K T H Consulting
Business Address ————— **Contact information**
Business Phone Number
Web Site Address

As a final check on form, remember the acronym SEND[1] to ensure that your message is simple (S), effective (E), necessary (N), and done (D) before you press the send button.

Beyond form, queries serve two functions. First, a good query sells your manuscript idea to an editor. To that end, a query is an "Ask" message[1] that establishes a relational connection with an editor. Your message establishes rapport through the tone in which you write and the respect that your message conveys. In their book on e-mail usage and protocol, Shipley and Schwalbe's two rules of etiquette apply: (1) Think before you send and (2) send mail you would like to receive.[1] The authors allow for the use of exclamation points and "emoticons," such as smiley faces.[1] Since my query is a formal request of a colleague with whom I have worked before, exclamation points seemed acceptable. I wouldn't include a smiley face, even though I do like and use them. A pleasant sign-off is the finishing touch before you include your name and contact information.

Second, queries serve as a writing sample for editors. A query is well written when every idea revolves around your slant/title *and* when the appeal of an idea for a vehicle's readership is made explicit. Notice in my query that I make the case for a third article about joy-stealing based on positive *RNL* reader response to the first two articles. As an editor, Jim's concern is that manuscript ideas and titles appeal to *RNL* readership.

In addition to brief queries like mine, there is a longer format that includes the following 10 items:[2]

1. Working title of manuscript that showcases your slant
2. Formal salutation (e.g., Dear Dr.)
3. Author's qualification to write on the topic
4. Brief description of the focused topic
5. Compelling description of why focused topic is important
6. Statement indicating familiarity with journal
7. Rationale for submitting to this journal/why this is an appealing topic for readership
8. Author's time frame for writing manuscript (optional)
9. A clear, well-written, well-organized writing style
10. Author's contact information

In preparation for translating her thesis into a manuscript, Kelly Rossler, a critical care nurse new to academe, completed the following worksheet.

Publication Worksheet

Name: Kelly L. Rossler   **My Product**: Journal Article

Idea: Human–Animal Bonding

   Topic: Effects of Animal Visitation on Hospice Patients

   Focus: Animal visitation as a therapeutic modality to reduce
        anxiety in terminally ill patients entering hospice facilities

Purpose: To educate hospice nurses about the documented effects of human–animal bonding and to move them to recommend animal visitation as a complementary treatment modality for hospice patients experiencing anxiety.

Audience: Oncology/Hospice Nurses

Venue/Vehicle: *Clinical Journal of Oncology Nursing*

Slant: From Bow-Wow to Meow: Pet Visitation Can Be a Hospice Patient's Best Friend

One-Sentence Description: This article will, in addition to demonstrating a need for nurses to conduct research in the realm of human-animal bonding, recommend animal visitation programs as a viable, complementary modality for hospice patients.

After developing her worksheet, it would be a full year before Kelly used this 10-item list as a guide to write the following query letter. Check whether Kelly's query includes all 10 items on the list for the longer query format.

Kelly's Query

RE: *From Bow-Wow to Meow: Pet Visitation Can Be a Hospice Patient's Best Friend*

May 10, 2007

Dear Mrs. Schnable:

While working on a concept-analysis paper, I became interested in the relationship between humans and animals, specifically that of human-animal bonding. Because patients diagnosed with a terminal illness may experience stressors that produce anxiety, my master's thesis research explored the impact of animal visitation on patient stress levels in a hospice facility.

Although my findings suggest that animal visitation can diminish patient anxiety, hospice nurses may not view animal visitation as a complementary approach for treating anxiety. In addition to demonstrating a need for nurses to conduct research in the realm of human-animal bonding, this manuscript recommends animal visitation programs as a viable, complementary modality for hospice patients.

Would you be interested in reviewing a manuscript for *Clinical Journal of Oncology Nursing* that describes how animal visitation can be effective in reducing anxiety in terminally ill patients admitted to hospice facilities? Thanks in advance for your kind response.

Sincerely,

Kelly L. Rossler, RN, MSN

University XXX
City/State
E-mail Address
Office Phone Number

Because Kelly received an affirmative response in 24 hours, it's clear that her query was effective in selling her manuscript idea to this editor. No wonder! Her query addresses an idea with appeal for the readership of this journal, has a snappy title that's descriptive and emotive, and is tightly organized around the focused topic and purpose identified in her publication worksheet. To make your query as appealing as it is easy to read, well organized, and compelling, plug your information into either the brief or the formal query format (Jot Box 63-1).

Jot Box 63-1

Your Query

_____

_____

_____

_____

_____

_____

_____

_____

_____

Should you decide to query editors, attending to both form and function increases the chances that they'll welcome reviewing your manuscript.

TIP
Work smart! Query editors to streamline your writing efforts.

References

1. Shipley, D., & Schwalbe, W. (2007). *SEND: The essential guide to email for office and home.* New York: Alfred A. Knopf.
2. Davidhizar, R. (1993, Fall). Elements of an effective query letter. *Nurse Author & Editor: A Newsletter for Nurse Authors, Reviewers, and Editors,* 3(4), 8–9.

What You Need to Know Before Querying Editors

Editors are people. They like to be treated with the same consideration and courtesy with which you would like to be treated.

Suzanne Hall Johnson

Writing your brief query outline at the end of Chapter 63 may have raised some general questions about queries for you. Excellent! Because query questions are so standard, this chapter poses nurses' most frequently asked questions and provides the answers.

Do All Editors Accept Queries?

No, but it's easy to find out which ones do. Most online descriptions of publications include a section called "Author Guidelines" that specifies whether editors accept queries. When this is not specified and the contact information for the editor or managing editor is provided, call or e-mail to ask about the advisability of submitting a query letter.

Why Don't All Editors Accept Queries?

Although queries may be working smart for authors, this isn't always true for editors. For example, Jim Mattson says, "Although I consider and have accepted articles on the basis of queries, I prefer manuscripts, as stated in *RNL*'s author guidelines, because they let me know for sure if an article is something I'm interested in." When authors do submit queries, Jim prefers that they be accompanied by a writing sample. For you, as an author, what's important is determining—if you choose to send queries—which editors accept queries.

Is a Query Always in the Form of an E-mail Message?

Not necessarily. Queries can also be made by phone. If you've met or been in contact with an editor previously, a phone contact works well. The same principle applies whether you're calling or e-mailing; editors are busy people and your job is to make their job as easy as possible. When phoning an editor, be prepared to give a succinct summary of your focused topic and why this appeals to the readership. In this case, use your query outline (Chapter 63) to prepare your summary statement. If you've never met the editor and this is your first time contacting him or her, I'd recommend an electronic query. Not only does this establish rapport and showcase your writing style, it allows editors to file your e-mail communication, organize communications, establish a paper trail, and track the editorial process.

How Many Queries Can I Send Out?

You can send as many as you want. This allows you to explore all possible vehicles and choose the ones, in order of priority, to write for. If you find one vehicle that seems perfect, that's great. If you find two or three possible vehicles, that's even better. Regarding turnaround time, I give editors 2 weeks to respond. If I haven't heard back by then, I resend my original e-mail message.

What if All Editors Queried Want to Review My Manuscript?

This is a delightful dilemma. First, thank the writing muse that your topic is intriguing enough to put the glitter in several editors' eyes. Then it's decision time. Because you can only submit one manuscript to a single editor, you have to choose. Once you commit to an editor, e-mail the other editors thanking them for their time. Explain that your query elicited a number of positive responses and that you've chosen the vehicle that seems the best fit. Leave the door open, because you never know what will happen with your first choice. It's perfectly acceptable to say that, should things not work out, you hope the editor would consider reviewing the manuscript for publication.

How Do You Make a Decision About Which Vehicle to Choose?

You may have been wondering how to prioritize your vehicles when you have several options. There are a number of reasons for choosing a particular vehicle:

1. Best source of information related to your topic
2. Prestige of journal in your specialty area
3. Widest readership, so your topic gets the greatest visibility
4. Refereed
5. Style of writing fits your writing style

Your choice depends on who you are, where you work, and what your reason is for publishing. Nurse entrepreneurs tend to be more interested in 3, because they're looking to reach the largest number of potential customers with their work. Nurse educators in a faculty positions will be most interested in 4, because most universities require that publications be refereed to count toward promotion and tenure. At this point in my career, 5 is most important to me. I only write for vehicles that accept informed-conversational style written in the first person.

What's a Refereed Publication?

A refereed publication is one in which manuscripts are reviewed by colleagues regarded as experts in the field. Editors send out manuscripts to between one and three reviewers who serve, without pay, as external reviewers. Editors make the final decision taking into account expert reviewers' recommendations as to the suitability of manuscripts based on criteria supplied by the vehicle. In the case of a nonrefereed vehicle, decisions to publish are made by one or two people, usually the editorial staff. Author guidelines specify whether a publication is refereed.

Will the Expert Reviewers Know Who I Am?

Sometimes yes and sometimes no. There are four types of review. With an *open review*, both the reviewer and the author are known to each other. With an *anonymous review*, the reviewer is not known to the author. With a *single-blind review*, the author is not known to the reviewer. With a *double-blind review*, neither editor nor author are known to the other. Sometimes a publication blends two approaches. For instance, *Nursing Education Perspectives* does an internal (anonymous) review where the author is known to the editors. If the manuscript is deemed acceptable for peer review, the manuscript is then sent without author identification to three external reviewers (double-blind review). Author guidelines often specify the type of review manuscripts undergo after being submitted.

What if I Don't Understand What an Editor's Response Means?

It happens. When a manuscript of mine was rejected for the third time, I was at the end of my rope. I knew the manuscript had merit, I just couldn't find an editor who agreed. That's when I called Suzanne Smith, the editor of *Nurse Educator*. When I read her the three rejection letters, she said the second rejection letter was actually an acceptance letter *if,* that is, I was willing to complete the requested revisions. No sooner had we gotten off the phone than I e-mailed the second editor to say I'd be more than happy to make the revisions. Even as a well-published author, I needed an expert editor to translate this editor's shorthand for acceptance-pending-revision. So never be afraid to ask if you're uncertain about an editor's response.

Now that you've read this chapter, you know what's needed to send your queries on their way. ▪

TIP

Work smart and e-mail queries to the editors of more than one periodical.

How to Rate an Editor's Response to Your Query

*The editor must serve and answer
first to the nursing readership.*

Joan Borgatti

Once you press the send button, an editor's response to your query is not far behind. Case in point, Jim Mattson's response to my query about my "joy-stealer is me" manuscript arrived within 24 hours after I sent it. Figure 65-1 shows the four potential editorial responses to queries.

Response	Level of Editorial Interest	
1. Reject	↑	None
2. Reject with recommendations for other possibilities		Low
3. Request to resubmit with different slant		
4. Request to review manuscript	↓	High

FIGURE 65-1   Potential Editorial Responses to Author Queries

As you read Jim's reply to my query, try and figure out which of the four fits his response.

Query Response

RE: What to Do When the Joy-Stealer is Me?

January 6, 2007

Jim Mattson wrote:

Hi Kathy,

Nice to hear from you. Nice also to learn that you have enough material for another article in the series.

Because of the time-connection to the previous articles about joy-stealing, I think it would fit well in the Third Qtr. 2007 issue, the theme of which is "Toward Reflective Practice." If my understanding of reflective practice is correct—taking time to look inward to find areas for self-improvement—an article titled "What happens when the joy-stealer is me?" would be right on target. Obviously, we would want to provide a bridge at the beginning of the article to alert readers who aren't aware of the previous articles of their existence. Copy deadline for that issue is July 20.

Sound like a plan?

Jim

James E. Mattson
Editor, *Reflections on Nursing Leadership (RNL)*

So where does Jim's response fit on the list of potential editorial responses? If you chose 4, I'd agree. Jim not only confirmed his interest in reviewing my manuscript, he accepted it sight unseen. The only reason this happened, and I'm glad it did, was that *RNL* reader interest was so strong in my two previous manuscripts on this topic.[1,2] Note also that Jim's response specified that the manuscript be written to relate to the theme of reflective practice. With this theme, Jim gave me the slant. What more could any author ask for?

Sad to say, it's not always a slam-dunk. In fact, if you're going to get into the publishing game, you may need to reframe the whole notion of rejection for yourself. Look at it this way. In an internal memo, a Knopf editor said of *The Bell Jar* by Sylvia Plath, "There certainly isn't enough genuine talent for us to take notice."[3] If writers become authors with their first rejection, then the sooner you get your own best rejection story, the better. Did I tell you about the time . . . Don't worry, I won't bore you with mine, but trust me, I've had more than my share of rejections. Back to reframing, when you consider that your ultimate goal is finding "the best home" for your manuscript, rejections are blessings in disguise. If not for rejections, you'd never find the right home for your manuscript.

With that said, the first type of rejection listed in Figure 65-1 is the toughest, because it's a flat refusal with no suggestions that point you in a new direction. The good news? You can cross this vehicle off your list and continue your search for a home. Can you imagine if you'd spent the time writing your manuscript and then submitted it to this editor who held it for six months and then rejected it?

The second editorial response carries you beyond the rejection by offering the names of editors and/or vehicles that might be interested in your topic. So while one door closes, this rejection response opens others.

The third editorial response is a strong indicator of editorial interest. When queries are resubmitted with a slant that's a better fit with the publication's readership, manuscripts have a good chance of being accepted for review. Your willingness to rework a slant will impress editors with your responsiveness, creativity, and perseverance.

The fourth response is the most exciting response for an author. Although a positive response to a query is not an acceptance of your manuscript, it is a sign of strong editorial interest. When you send out a number of queries and receive several positive responses, prioritize the "yes we're interested" vehicles in order of your preference. Submit your manuscript to the first vehicle on your vehicle list. Should that manuscript be rejected, you've got your second and third options all lined up. Having multiple options puts a whole new spin on rejection.

TIP

Make sure you understand an editor's response to your query before you make your next move.

References

1. Heinrich, K. T. (2006, Third Quarter). Joy-stealing: How some nurse educators resist these faculty games. *Reflections on Nursing Leadership.* Retrieved August 21, 2007, from http://nursingsociety.org/RNL/3Q_2006/features/feature6.html
2. Heinrich, K. T. (2006, Second Quarter). Joy-stealing games. *Reflections on Nursing Leadership.* Retrieved August 21, 2007, from http://www.nursing-society.org/RNL/2Q_2006/features/feature5.html
3. Max, T. (2007, June 11, 18). Final destination: Letter from Austin. *The New Yorker,* p. 64.

What You Need to Proceed with Your Writing Project

I shall become a master in this art only after a great deal of practice.

Erich Fromm

Let's pause to gather the worksheets you'll need to complete the rest of the Strategies and Skills chapters. Because nothing in this chapter is new to you, this is going to be a see-mine, complete-yours sequence. The first step is finalizing your Publication Worksheet. See my completed worksheet for the "joy-stealer is me" writing project.

Publication Worksheet

Idea: Joy-stealing

> **Topic:** Competitive games played by nurse educators that steal joy

> **Focus:** What happens when the joy-stealer is me?

Purpose: My purpose in writing up what I learned from the participants in the joy-stealing workshop is *to inform* readers about how

(continues)

Publication Worksheet

nurse educators report stealing each other's joy as well as *to move* them to examine their own behavior as joy stealers.

Readers: Academic nurses

Vehicle: *Reflections on Nursing Leadership (RNL)*

Desired Reader Response: Learn from colleagues' reflections on being joy-stealers and reflect on how they, the readers, steal other's joy.

Slant (Title): Reflective Practice

One-Sentence Description: This article will share stories from nurse educators that describe the ways they steal joy and suggest strategies for stopping the joy-stealing.

To double-check that my items are logically developed and flow from one another, we'll complete the same Three-Question Quiz we used for the Presentation Worksheet (Section II, Chapter 21):

Three-Question Quiz

1. Does vehicle fit readership? **Yes ☑ No ☐**

   My Vehicle: Professional magazine targeting nurse educators

   My Readership: Nurse educators

2. Does purpose fit desired reader response? **Yes ☑ No ☐**

   My Purpose: To teach, to motivate to action

   Desired Reader Response: Learn, move to action

3. Does slant include a descriptive and an emotive component?
   Yes ☐ No ☑

   Because my slant is not yet a title, I checked no.

Feel free to tweak the items as you transcribe the information from your Presentation Worksheet to the worksheet provided here.

Publication Worksheet

Idea: _____

_____

Topic: _____

Focus: _____

Purpose: _____

Readership: _____

Vehicle: _____

Desired Reader Response: _____

Slant (Title): _____

One-sentence description: This article will _____

Complete the Three-Question Quiz on the next page to ensure that your items hang together.

When you're satisfied with your answers, take a look at the Kolb-It Worksheet design for my 15-minute presentation and PowerPoint slide display titled "The Joy-Stealer Is Me."

Three-Question Quiz

1. Does vehicle fit readership? **Yes** ❑ **No** ❑

   Your Vehicle: _____

   Your Readers: _____

2. Does purpose fit desired reader response? **Yes** ❑ **No** ❑

   Your Purpose: _____

   Your Desired Reader Response: _____

3. Does slant include a descriptive and an emotive component?

   Yes ❑ **No** ❑

Kolb-It Worksheet

My Presentation Title: The Joy Stealer is Me!

CE: *Vignette*: How a nurse stole a colleague's joy

Free-write: Write about a time when you said or did something that stole a student's, colleague's, or administrator's joy.

RO: What was it like for you to write about this?

AC:

Slide #1

Joy-Stealing

Experiences with students, colleagues, staff, and administrators that rob nurse educators of their zest, clarity, productivity, feelings of worth, and desire for more connection.[2]

(continues)

Kolb-It Worksheet (continued)

Slide #2

Stop projecting blame onto others.

Start owning "shadow" qualities.[3]

Slide #3

Undertake a "personal growth agenda to confront our own shadow, heal our wounds, and become self-authoring and self-transforming."[3]

Slide #4

Renew our commitment to a scholarship of reflective practice.[3]

Slide #5

Keep a Teacher's Notebook

    1. Own my own shortcomings.

    2. Deepen compassion for others' shortcomings.

    3. Become my own ally.

AE: *Free-write*: How has seeing myself as a joy-stealer influenced my perspective on joy-stealing?

RO: *Affirmation*: Knowing what I know now, my next step in facing the joy-stealer within is . . .

Now it's your turn to insert the information on your Kolb-It Design Worksheet from Chapter 35 into Jot Box 66-1.

Jot Box 66-1

Your Presentation Kolb-It Design

CE: _____

RO: _____

AC: _____

AE: _____

RO: _____

With your worksheets completed, you're ready to create a timeline to keep you on schedule. Before you do, if you have not done so already, translate the information from your completed Publication Worksheet to Appendix C and Kolb-It Design Worksheet to Appendix B so you can use them in completing the exercises in the rest of this Strategies and Skills section.

TIP

Keeping your worksheets in front of you will help you stay true to your original idea.

References

1. Clark, C., & Heinrich, K. T. (2007, January). *Cultivating civility in nursing education: From today's realities to tomorrow's possibilities.* Pre-conference Workshop, Mosby's Faculty Development Institute, San Diego, CA.
2. Heinrich, K. T. (2007). Joy stealing. 10 mean games faculty play and how to stop the gaming. *Nurse Educator, 32*(1), 34–38.
3. Pesut, D. (2004). Creating the future through renewal: 2003–2005 presidential call to action. *Reflections on Nursing Leadership, 30*(1), 24.

What to Consider as You Craft Your Timeline

67

Don't fail to make your deadline.

Joan Borgatti

Writing projects, like presenting projects, go more smoothly when you design a timeline that fits your schedule and delivers your product to your editor on time.[1] A timeline ensures that you identify the tasks involved in preparing your manuscript for publication and allocate enough time to attend to them. As in Chapter 66, you're adapting a strategy you learned in Section II to fit your publication project, so this is another see-one, do-one chapter. I used a timeline to keep my "joy-stealer is me" writing project on track.

The first date I wrote is Jim's deadline—July 20—and I worked back from that date to develop my timeline. My list is relatively short. Note that I didn't include time to search for a vehicle, because I'd already determined the vehicle. Nor did I do a literature search because mine was only 4 months old, and it's standard practice to leave 6 months between searches.

My Timeline for the Joy-Stealing Manuscript

Task	Time Frame
1. Compose query to *RNL* editor	January 5
2. Receive acceptance	January 6
3. Complete Publication Worksheet	March 14
4. Complete timeline	March 14
5. Free-write/mind map/outline ideas	April 1
6. Translate Kolb-It Worksheet into manuscript	April 10
7. Write shitty first draft (SFD)	April 15
8. Choose and contact peer editors	May 15
9. Send SFD to peer editors	June 1
10. Revise SFD with peer editors' feedback	June 10
11. Send manuscript draft to *RNL* editor	June 17
12. Revise final draft for *RNL* with editor's feedback	June 25
13. Submit final draft to *RNL* editor	July 1
14. *RNL* copy deadline	July 20

Here's a list of tasks to consider adding to your timeline depending upon your preferences as an author and the requirements of your writing project:

1. Locate an eye-glittering idea.
2. Complete the Publication Worksheet.
3. Identify potential vehicles.
4. Compose queries.
5. Choose peer editor(s).
6. Ask peer editor(s) to review query.
7. Create a list of potential vehicles based on editorial responses.
8. Free-write/mind map/outline ideas.
9. Divide outline into 15-minute chunks.
10. Write shitty first draft (SFD).
11. Send SFD to peer editor(s).
12. Revise SFD with peer editor(s') feedback.
13. Submit revised manuscript.
14. Celebrate!

15. If rejected, use editorial feedback to revise and send to next vehicle on list.
16. If revision is required for acceptance, revise ASAP, and return to editors with itemized list of responses to editorial feedback.
17. If accepted as is, enjoy the glow!
18. Celebrate!

The more specific the tasks, the longer the to-do list, the longer the timeline. Add as many items as needed; the number of items makes no difference. For example, you may want to divide your writing projects into three tasks that each carry a completion date—beginning, middle, and end. Short or long, detailed or general, make your time frames reasonable and achievable. Because I always underestimate the time writing projects take, I add a week onto any estimate of mine. Complete the following timeline to keep you and your project on target.

Your Timeline	
Task	**Time Frame**
1. Complete publication worksheet	(Today's Date)
2. _____	_____
3. _____	_____
4. _____	_____
5. _____	_____
6. _____	_____
7. _____	_____
	(continues)

Your Timeline (continued)	
Task	**Time Frame**
8. _____	_____
9. _____	_____
10. _____	_____
11. _____	_____
12. _____	_____
13. _____	_____
14. _____	_____
15. _____	_____
16. _____	_____
17. _____	_____
18. _____	_____
19. _____	_____
20. _____	_____

Make it easier to locate the timeline you just constructed by transferring the task and time frame items into the "Timeline Worksheet for Publications" in Appendix D. Do revisit your timeline p.r.n. and make changes when phases go more quickly or more slowly than you anticipate. In the next chapters, you will free-write, mind-map, and outline your ideas and access peer editors. Once you know what each of these tasks involves, you may want to amend your timeline.

> **TIP**
>
> Keep your timeline detailed enough to keep you on track and flexible enough to serve as a guide rather than a straitjacket.

References

1. Oermann, M. H. (1999). Extensive writing projects: Tips for completing them on time. *Nurse Author & Editor, 9*(1), 8–10.

How to Tell if You're a Free-Writer, a Mind-Mapper, or an Outliner

68

*Divide your writing task into
15-minute blocks of time.*

Suzanne Hall Johnson

Outlining is the proper way to organize ideas for writing projects. True or false? It's both. Even though we all learned to outline our papers in school, when it comes to organizing ideas there is no right or wrong. The reality is that each of us starts writing projects in our own way. So don't be afraid to be honest. When you have a writing assignment, how do you begin?

Jot Box 68-1

❑ a. Sit down and start writing.

❑ b. Place your idea in the center of a paper and scribble all the related ideas you can think of around it.

❑ c. Create an outline.

❑ d. Other. _____

Whether you know it or not, you've just chosen one of three possible approaches for organizing your ideas for writing projects—free-writing, mind-mapping, and outlining. Compare your answer with mine.

When I have a writing assignment, how do I begin?

☑ a. Sit down and start writing. [*Free-writer*]

❑ b. Place your idea in the center of a paper and scribble all the related ideas you can think of around it. [*Mind-mapper*]

❑ c. Create an outline. [*Outliner*]

❑ d. Other. _____

If you chose option a, then you start a writing project with a free-write. If you picked option b, then you're a mind-mapper who grabs a piece of paper, writes your idea in the center of the page, and scribbles every idea or concept you can think of around that central idea. Then you cluster separate ideas into themes. If you chose option c, then you're an outliner.

After years of teaching nurses how to write for publication, I've learned that mind-mappers and outliners come from different planets. Outliners get dizzy when they see ideas splattered all over a piece of paper. Mind-mappers' jaws clench at the thought of squeezing the juice out of creative ideas by smushing them into grids neatly labeled with Roman numerals. The only ones not fazed by either mind-mapping or outlining are free-writers. I suspect this has to do with the fact that they use all three approaches. That said, there's no reason you have to choose just one option; it's possible to use each of these three approaches sequentially. Let me show you by using the "joy-stealer is me" example. I start with a free-write.

The "Joy-stealer Is Me" Free-Write

I want to make good on my promise to get our Mosby workshop participants' stories published. I'm so glad I queried Jim Mattson because writing a manuscript for *RNL* is a double gift. I can write my manuscript in an informed-conversational style in the first person. Not only is this my favorite writing style, but this is the style that allows me to stay true to participants' stories. An added bonus is writing for an editor like Jim who makes the process easy with his clear expectations and quick turnaround time.

When I looked back at my presentation, I was relieved to see how much of the work was already done. Because of my literature search, I'm able to use Daniel Pesut's ideas to link to the slant of reflective practice. Since Daniel Pesut was then the President of Sigma Theta Tau, the organization that publishes *RNL*, readers will be interested in how his ideas apply to joy-stealing.

I still need to reread participants' free-writes from the "joy-stealer is me" workshop presentation to pick out the themes. After analyzing the data, I'll know if the one-sentence description on my Publication Worksheet needs reworking, "This article is written to help readers explore how they steal joy from students, colleagues and administrators; to deepen their compassion for joy-stealers; and to initiate dialogues about joy-stealing in faculty meetings, classrooms and clinical settings."

Notice how this free-write allowed me to reflect on my feelings about this project, as well as to brainstorm ideas for proceeding with the actual writing process, both of which are tasks related to developing this manuscript.

My second step is mind-mapping. You've probably heard of *concept mapping,* which allows nurses ". . . to synthesize relevant data such as diagnoses, signs and symptoms, health needs, nursing interventions, and assessments."[1] A *mind map* is an older term that extends the meaning of concept maps beyond clinical applications. Mind maps are visual representations that organize and synthesize information so that complex relationships between and among ideas, concepts, and theories can be understood.[2] The following mind map is a combination of items from my Publication Worksheet (Chapter 62), my Kolb-It Design (Chapter 66), and my analysis of the stories gathered from the Mosby workshop participants (see Figure 68-1).

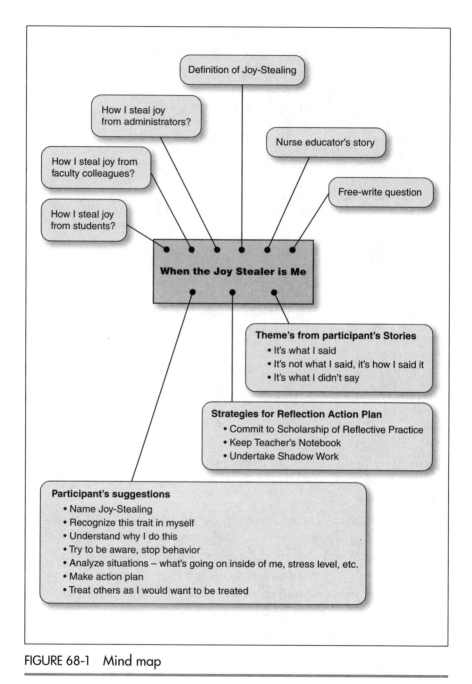

FIGURE 68-1   Mind map

My mind map allows me to visualize the relationships between and among the ideas and concepts that revolve around my slant. From this visual, I construct an outline.[1] For me, the easiest way to begin to translate a mind map into an outline for a manuscript is to separate the manuscript draft into three sections—beginning, middle, and end. Beginnings are said to be the implicit promise, middles develop that promise, and endings deliver on the promise.

Outline

Working Title of Manuscript: The Full-Circle Moment: Recognizing the Joy-Stealer in Me

I. BEGINNING
   A. Opening Quotation [Find]
   B. Introduction [15 minutes]
      1. Connect this article with past two articles on joy-stealing
      2. Participants share stories of their stealing other's joy
      3. One-sentence description (Presentation Worksheet)

II. MIDDLE
   A. What happened at the Conference [15 minutes]
      1. Joy-stealing Defined
      2. Nurse Educator's Story
      3. Free-write Question Posed
   B. Themes from Stories Collected [several hours of 15-minute blocks]
   C. Definition of Reflective Practice (Daniel Pesut)
   D. Suggestions from Participants
   E. Strategies for Reflective Action Plan [several hours of 15-minute blocks]

III. ENDING [15 minutes after the rest of steps are completed.]
   A. Summary
   B. Conclusion

Can you see how each of these three general sections divides into 15-minute writing assignments (e.g., finding the best definition for reflective practice)? Depending on how many 15-minute chunks open up in my schedule, this manuscript might be finished up within a couple of days or weeks with a few polishing sessions thrown in before I send my shitty first draft to my peer editor.

Decide which strategy or strategies you'll use to organize the ideas and concepts from your Publication and Kolb-It Worksheets into an outline. I'll leave that creative task to you, whether you're a free-writer, mind-mapper, or outliner, or a bit of all three. You may want to use your *Dare to Share* notebook as the repository for your organizational musings. And, now that you've seen how all three strategies work, don't be afraid to play with the ones you've never tried out before. You may delight yourself by discovering a new way or a new combination of ways to organize your ideas.

TIP

Use free-writing, mind-mapping, and outlining to focus your ideas around your slant for writing projects.

References

1. King, M., & Shell, R. (2002). Teaching and evaluating critical thinking with concept maps. *Nurse Educator, 27*(50), 214–216.
2. Hill, C. M. (2006, January/February). Integrating clinical experiences into the concept mapping process. *Nurse Educator, 31*(1), 36–39.
3. Oermann, M. H. (2000). Refining outlining skills: Part 1: The topic or sentence method. *Nurse Author & Editor, 10*(2), 4, 7–8.

How to Leap from Outlines to Manuscripts

69

Your job as an author is to make your editor's job easy. Follow directions to the letter.

Suzanne Hall Johnson

As reassuring as it is to have an outline, are you feeling a bit unsure about how to turn your outline into the publishable product? No wonder, this is a creative leap, and leaping from the known to the unknown is always good for making the heart pound a little faster. To show you how to make this creative leap, this chapter follows the steps I used in translating my outline for the "joy-stealer is me" project into a manuscript. Author guidelines, as well as your Publication Worksheet and Kolb-It Design Worksheet, can help you bridge the known and unknown.

When it comes to developing your manuscript from your outline, use author guidelines and directions set out by the editor and the publication as a guide. In addition to the *RNL* "Instructions for Authors" available at the Sigma Theta Tau International Honor Society's Web site, I made a list of directions that I received from Jim Mattson in e-mail messages. Notes to myself are italicized:

1. **Word count**. 1300 to 1500 words. *Follow requirements for margins and font size and stay within word limitations.*
2. **Informed-conversational style**. Jim says, "I like articles that communicate directly with the reader." *Write in first person, informed-conversational style.*

297

3. **The theme of the issue.** In this case, the theme for the issue is "Toward Reflective Practice." *Make reflective practice my slant.*

4. **Link to previous articles.** Jim said, "we would want to provide a bridge at the beginning of the article to alert readers who aren't aware of the previous articles of their existence." *Will do.*

5. **Focused topic**: What to Do When the Joy-Stealer Is Me

6. **The Slant (Title)**: The Full Circle Moment: Recognizing the Joy-Stealer in Me. *Both the full-circle moment and recognizing refer to reflective practice.*

7. **Time frame.** Copy deadline is July 20. *I plan to set deadlines for Jim to review earlier drafts so I have my final version to him well before his deadline.*

8. **Publication format:** APA

9. **Revision policy**: While authors review manuscripts after editorial review, I understand that my title and text may be altered by the editor prior to publication.

If you nail the introduction, the manuscript will write itself. That's why I've chosen to share the introduction from the manuscript I am submitting to *RNL* to illustrate how easily a well-conceptualized outline translates into a manuscript draft along with the heading for the middle and my approach to writing conclusions.

Manuscript Draft

The Full-Circle Moment: Recognizing the Joy-Stealer in Me

[This title is in keeping with the theme of Reflective Practice.]

Kathleen T. Heinrich, RN, PhD

BEGINNING

> Compassion is not a relationship between the healer and the wounded. It's a relationship between equals. Only when we know our own darkness well can we be present with the darkness of others. Compassion becomes real when we recognize our shared humanity.
> —Pema Chödrön

(continues)

[If you like to open with a quotation, make sure that it resonates with and amplifies your slant. In my case, nurses who undertake the difficult challenge of looking at the joy stealer within need to be compassionate toward themselves.]

It's one thing to talk about times when you've had your joy stolen by students, colleagues or administrators. It's a whole other thing to admit to being the one who steals joy from others. *[You've got to grab your reader in the first two sentences so make sure they're intriguing, surprising or beguiling enough to make this happen.]* That's why I wasn't sure how willing nurse educators would be to talk about themselves as joy-stealers. Twenty-five courageous and introspective nurse educators at the Mosby Faculty Institute not only shared their stories with each other, they gave me permission to share their stories with you (Clark & Heinrich, 2007). *[Give your readers enough of a context so they know what you're talking about but don't try to tell them everything in the introductory section.]*

As a follow-up to two articles that explored how students, faculty colleagues, and administrators steal our joy as nurse educators (Heinrich, 2006, Heinrich 2006a) *[This is the "bridge" Jim requested be made to previous two articles.]*, this article shares how 25 educators say they stole students, colleagues, and administrators' joy, describes "full circle moments" when telling on themselves increases educators' compassion for joy-stealers and joy stealing, and shares suggestions for reflective practice. *[In your introduction, tell readers how the chapter is organized. This orients them and invites them to follow along.]*

MIDDLE

[Make sure to stay consistent. Whatever your introductory sentence promises to be covered becomes the headings for the various sections in the body of your manuscript.]

How Nurse Educators Steal Joy

Full-Circle Moments

Suggestions for Reflective Practice

END

Summary

Conclusion

[For me, the conclusion will be the last thing I write after revising this manuscript based on peer editor's reviews. My conclusion will reiterate my slant/title—The Full-Circle Moment: Recognizing the Joy-Stealer in Me.]

As you can see, it's taken very little effort to move from my outline to a manuscript draft. Although the time spent completing the Publication Worksheet and organizing ideas into free-writes, mind-maps, and outlines may seem excessive, when it comes to manuscript-writing time, the work is pretty much done. If you're curious to see what it looks like in final form, you can access the published article by going to the *Reflections on Nursing Leadership* magazine posted on Sigma Theta Tau International's Web site. Either go to the honor society's home page www.nursingsociety.org and click on the link provided there or go directly to www.nursingsociety.org/ RNL/3Q_2007/index.html.

This chapter ends the Strategies and Skills portion of this section. The rest of this section is devoted to the relational dimension of writing projects, called "support circles." Just as you learned to craft conscious relationships with co-presenters and collaborators on presentation projects, the same goes for co-authors and collaborators on writing projects.

In concluding this portion of this section, I'd like to formally acknowledge Jim Mattson's contributions; to thank him for the time and care he took with reviewing Chapters 61, 62, 65, 66, 67, and 70; and to thank him for his thought-provoking questions and insightful suggestions that so improved them.

TIP

Work smart! Use your writing time efficiently by organizing your ideas up-front.

References

1. Heinrich, K. T. (2006, Second Quarter). Joy-stealing games. *Reflections on Nursing Leadership*. Retrieved August 21, 2007, from http://www.nursing-society.org/RNL/2Q_2006/features/feature5.html
2. Heinrich, K. T. (2006, Third Quarter). Joy-stealing: How some nurse educators resist these faculty games. *Reflections on Nursing Leadership*. Retrieved August 21, 2007, from http://nursingsociety.org/RNL/3Q_2006/features/feature6.html
3. Clark, C., & Heinrich, K. T. (2007, January). *Cultivating civility in nursing education: From today's realities to tomorrow's possibilities.* Pre-conference Workshop, Mosby's Faculty Development Institute, San Diego, CA.
4. Heinrich, K. T. (2007). Joy-stealing. 10 mean games faculty play and how to stop the gaming. *Nurse Educator, 32*(1), 34–38.

How to Think Like an Editor When Preparing Your Manuscript

70

Editors are people too! Treat them with the same courtesy with which you would like to be treated.

Suzanne Hall Johnson

Just as nurse-authors have a favorite rejection story, they also have favorite stories about a particular editor's generosity and encouragement. Mine goes back to a chilly Wednesday in November, the day before Thanksgiving, when a phone call interrupted a nap tucked between cleaning the house and making cranberry relish. Still half asleep, I finally realized the caller was an editor saying how moved she was by the nurses' experiences described in my manuscript. She had had some of the same experiences, and even though she couldn't use the piece in her journal she mentioned the names of a few editors who might be interested. The fact that she took the time to call was so exhilarating that I barely noticed that she'd rejected my query request. Her affirmation carried me through the query process to find the perfect home for that manuscript.

Experiences like this one have taught me that the best editors serve the interests of their readers *and* mentor new authors. As with all colleagues, authors' relationships with editors grow naturally out of working together on publishing projects. To show you how true this is, I asked five editors who've mentored me over the years, along with one review editor, to share their do's, don'ts, and "must reads." Even though you may not have noticed, quotations from them are sprinkled throughout the Strategies & Skills chapters you've just read. These editors and reviewers for nursing newsletters, magazines, and journals include:

> Joan Borgatti, RN, MEd, Editor Emeritus, *NURSING Spectrum New England*
>
> Peggy Chinn, RN, PhD, FAAN, Editor, *Advances in Nursing Science*
>
> Suzanne Hall Johnson, RN, MN, CNS, Editor Emeritus, *Nurse Author & Editor: A Newsletter for Nurse Authors, Reviewers, and Editors and Dimensions of Critical Care Nursing*
>
> Melinda Granger Oberleitner, RN, DNS, APRN, CNS, Member of Editorial Review Board, *Oncology Nursing Forum*
>
> Marilyn H. Oermann, RN, PhD, FAAN, Editor, *Journal of Nursing Care Quality*
>
> Suzanne Smith, RN, EdD, FAAN, Editor, *Nurse Educator* and *Journal of Nursing Administration*

Summed up in three words, their advice is this*: Think like editors*. As Joan Borgatti points out:

> Editors must serve and answer first to their nursing readership and it is with that particular viewpoint that they review authors' submissions. When editors are under the gun and swamped by paperwork, only the great stuff gets noticed. The rest gets barely a read-through before it is sentenced to the circular file. So make sure to tell editors in your queries how a manuscript fits their readership; make sure manuscripts fit their journal's mission, format and writing style.

To start thinking like an editor, take a look at the points on which these editors agree.

Do's for Nurse-Authors

- Narrow your topic to a specific focus or slant.
- Write for readers. Ask what they'd want to know about your topic.
- Identify possible periodicals; submit to the top one on your list first.

- Write your manuscript *for* this periodical.
- Review the last 1 to 2 years of volumes.
- Use an article with a topic and writing style similar to yours as a guide.
- Consider the "Author Guidelines" as a road map to a great article.
- Give the editor everything he/she asks for—and then some.
- Ask a colleague(s) with publication experience to peer edit your manuscript.
- Give your peer editor(s) enough time to provide a thoughtful review.
- Proof carefully before sending.
- Ask the editor when in doubt.
- Take a rejection or a revision request as an opportunity to press forward.

Don'ts for Nurse-Authors

- Don't write a manuscript and then look for a possible journal.
- Don't write about a topic that's been well published without a fresh slant.
- Don't submit a manuscript to an editor on a topic he/she just published.
- Don't submit a "school paper" to a journal. Editors can tell.
- Don't submit your first draft.
- Don't stalk the editor! Nothing turns off an editor like daily phone calls.
- Don't make readers hunt for your idea in long, intricate paragraphs.
- Don't publish the same message more than once.
- Don't write more than one or two articles about the same project.
- Don't submit a co-authored piece until it reads like one author wrote it.
- Don't overdo figures and tables.
- Don't make careless formatting, grammatical, or spelling mistakes.
- Don't fail to make your deadline(s).
- Don't submit a rejected manuscript to a new periodical without revising.

"Must Reads" for Nurse-Authors

Do you want practical advice from nurse-authors and editors on timely topics? The publication that got the most editors' votes for a "must read" was the periodical initiated by Suzanne Hall Johnson called *Nurse Author & Editor: A Newsletter For Nurse Authors, Reviewers, and Editors.* Now available online, this newsletter is edited by Christine Webb.[1]

For basic texts on writing, they recommended two old standby's: *Chicago Manual of Style*[2] and *The Elements of Style.*[3] If you're in the market for an uplifting alternative, purchase a copy of *The Elements of Style Illustrated.*[4] Speaking of fun reads on an unlikely topic, there's a bestseller by a British woman named Lynn Truss called *Eats, Shoots and Leaves: The Zero-Tolerance Approach to Punctuation.*[5] On a similar note, if you've never read books about writing by creative writers you should treat yourself to Natalie Goldberg's *Writing Down the Bones*[6] and Anne Lamont's *Bird by Bird.*[7]

For those wanting to learn more about publishing in nursing, several editors also recommended Marilyn Oermann's textbook *Writing for Publication in Nursing.*[8] If you're interested in learning more about the rules of the road, Suzanne Smith suggests that ". . . the best resource for a quick overview of ethics related to writing for publication is a pithy document titled 'Problems with Writing a Paper,'"[9] which discusses the following:

- Not using other people's words or data (plagiarism)
- Not reporting contradictory observations you made
- Not putting your name on work you didn't do
- Not reporting others' related or contradictory work
- Not changing the hypothesis for the paper
- Not gradually changing from "far out possibility" to "established fact"
- Not concluding "cause and effect" when only "correlation" is demonstrated
- Not writing an abstract without including data
- Not reporting negative results
- Not publishing the same results many times
- Not allowing review of the manuscript or obtaining approval from all authors

Those of you seeking guidance for publishing research findings in a reader-friendly way would do well to track down Oermann et al.'s article in *Nurse Researcher*[10] and Tornquist's book *From Proposal to Publication: An Informal Guide to Writing About Nursing Research.*[11]

Follow the advice of these six editors, along with their recommendations for resources and references, and you're well on your way to getting published.

I would like to formally acknowledge Joan Borgatti, Peggy Chinn, Suzanne Hall Johnson, Melinda Oberleitner, Marilyn Oermann, and Suzanne Smith for their contributions to this chapter that reflect the good sense, good humor, and good will, not to mention generosity, which they have shown me over the years.

TIP
Relationships with editors grow out of your working together.

References

1. *Nurse Author and Editor* [Online]. Available at www.nurseauthoreditor.com
2. The University of Chicago. (2006, 2007). *Chicago manual of style online* (15th ed.). Retrieved September 7, 2007, from http://www.chicagomanualofstyle.org/home.html
3. Strunk, W., White, E. B., & Angell, R. (1999). *The elements of style* (4th ed.). Boston: Allyn & Bacon.
4. Strunk, W., White, E. B., & Kalman, M. (2005). *The elements of style illustrated.* New York: Penguin Press.
5. Truss, L. (2003). *Eats, shoots and leaves: The zero-tolerance approach to punctuation.* New York: Gotham Books.
6. Goldberg, N. (1986). *Writing down the bones: Freeing the writer within.* Boston: Shambala Productions, Inc.
7. Lamont, A. (1994). *Bird by bird: Some instructions on writing and life.* New York: First Anchor Books.
8. Oermann, M. H. (2002). *Writing for publication in nursing.* Philadelphia: Lippincott, Williams & Wilkins.
9. Mann, M. D. (n.d.). *Problems with writing a paper.* Retrieved September 7, 2007, from http://www.unmc.edu/ethics/data/data_wri.htm
10. Oermann, M. H., Galvin, E. A., Floyd, J. A., & Roop, J. C. (2006). Presenting research to clinicians: Strategies for writing about research findings. *Nurse Researcher, 13*(4), 66–74.
11. Tornquist, E. M. (1999). *From proposal to publication: An informal guide to writing about nursing research.* Menlo Park, CA: Addison-Wesley.

How to Choose Peer Editors and Request Peer Editing

71

Ask and ye shall receive.

The Bible

While everyone has heard of editors, many nurses who publish frequently aren't quite sure what a peer editor does. A *peer editor* is a colleague whom authors ask to review their written work, from queries through final drafts. According to Suzanne Hall Johnson, there are three types of peer editors: expert, general audience, and style. An *expert editor* is a colleague with expertise in the author's topic area. A *general audience editor* is a colleague who represents the author's readership. A *style editor* is anyone—a colleague or even a family member—familiar with the intricacies of grammar and punctuation. To this, I've added another category: *developmental peer editors*. Such peer editors help authors develop their presentations into publications and guide them in the publication process from query to acceptance. Such editors may or may not be nurses.

Approaching a peer editor before you know what you need is like expecting a waiter to know what you want for dinner without your order. So how do you figure out what you need? Responding to the following questionnaire helped me to clarify what types of peer editing I needed to prepare my manuscript.

Peer Editing Requirements Checklist

My Next Writing Task: When the Joy-Stealer Is Me

1. **What type(s) of editor does my writing task need:**

   ✔ a. Expert in specialty area

   ✔ b. Audience

   ✔ c. Style/mechanics

      d. Developmental

2. **Which colleague(s) can serve as an:**

   a. Expert Editor: Cindy Clark, Susan Luparell

   b. General Audience Editor: Christina Purpora

   c. Style Editor: Christina Purpora

3. **What style of feedback do I want:**

   a. Only positive (+)

   b. Only what's wrong (–)

   ✔ c. Positive and constructively critical feedback (+,–)

As you can see, I ended up with a list of three colleagues and the roles I wanted to ask them to take as peer editors. I chose Drs. Cindy Clark and Susan Luparell because they are expert researchers in incivility and Christina Purpora because she is conducting her doctoral research in incivility and she is an experienced peer editor, having peer edited *Dare to Share*.

Now it's time for you to get specific about your peer editing needs.

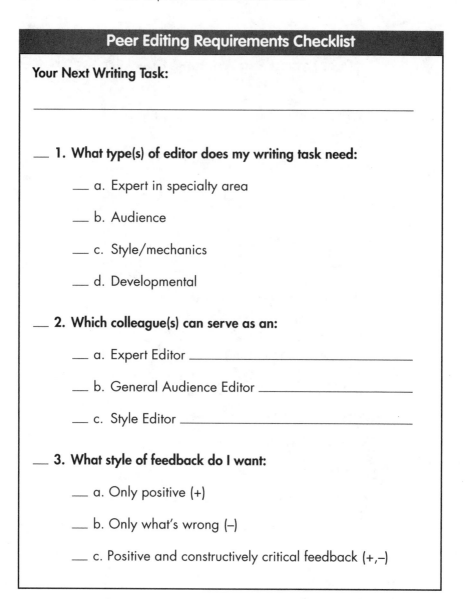

Peer Editing Requirements Checklist

Your Next Writing Task:

_____

___ **1. What type(s) of editor does my writing task need:**

    ___ a. Expert in specialty area

    ___ b. Audience

    ___ c. Style/mechanics

    ___ d. Developmental

___ **2. Which colleague(s) can serve as an:**

    ___ a. Expert Editor _____

    ___ b. General Audience Editor _____

    ___ c. Style Editor _____

___ **3. What style of feedback do I want:**

    ___ a. Only positive (+)

    ___ b. Only what's wrong (–)

    ___ c. Positive and constructively critical feedback (+,–)

At best, you've named several colleagues who might be willing to serve as peer editors. At worst, you're now on the look out for colleagues who fit the bill.

Once you've identified colleagues as potential peer editors, it's time to contact them. Taking my preferences into account allowed me to write the following request to Cindy Clark:

Request for Peer Editing

Re. *The Full-Circle Moment:* ———— **Title of manuscript**
Recognizing the Joy-Stealer in Me

Dear Cindy: ——**Greeting**

/**Rationale for Request**

Hope all is well! I'm writing to ask a favor. Knowing
you were as moved as I was by our workshop participants' stories about how they stole other's joy, I
wanted to ask your kindness in reviewing a manuscript
that shares these stories.

/**Request for Expert Editor**

Given your expertise on incivility in nursing education,
your editing suggestions would be particularly valuable.

/**Time Frame**

Jim Mattson has accepted this manuscript for publication in the third Quarter of *RNL*. Since the manuscript
is brief—between 1300-1500 words—I'd ask that your
feedback be returned within a week after you receive
the manuscript.

/**Reward**

Your editing of this manuscript will be acknowledged in
the published article. Please let me know if you're
interested and we'll go from there.

/**Closing**

Many thanks for your consideration,

Kathy

As you can see from the opening paragraph, I wrote Cindy first,
because, in addition to being an expert in incivility research, she was my
co-presenter at the session where I collected the "joy-stealer is me" stories. The labels on my "Ask" e-mail indicate that this message fits the
form for such inquiries:

- Request the favor of peer editing.
- Specify the type of manuscript and type of editorial feedback
  desired.
- Define a time frame and designate a turnaround time.

It's important to tell potential peer editors what's in it for them to peer edit your work. The best way to reward peer editors for their time is to formally acknowledge their contribution in the publication.

Now that you know what you want, it's time to compose a formal request(s) for peer editing. Make each message personal, tell your potential peer editors how much time it will take, specify your preference for a turnaround time, and thank them for considering your request. In the next chapter, you'll see what an entire cycle of peer editing looks like from invitation to thank you note.

TIP

The clearer you are about what you're asking of your peer editors, the more likely you are to get it.

How to Request, Respond to, and Reward Peer Editing

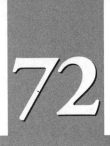

It's rare that we truly meet one another. If you can sense the inner body when you're facing someone, and remain in stillness without judging—just a feeling of presence—then you've truly met that human being.

Eckhart Tolle

When Lisa Nowak confirmed her interest in my writing an article for the school nurses' newsletter, I contacted my colleague–friend Christina to ask if she would be interested in peer editing my manuscript:

```
        Formal Request for Peer Editing

Re: Joy Stealing: What CT School Nurses Taught Me About
    Stopping the Game Playing [Working Title]


Dear Christina: [Salutation]
Hope all is well! I'm writing to ask your kindness in
peer editing a short manuscript on joy-stealing for a
newsletter. [Form of Manuscript]
```
(continues)

```
I'd like your feedback as an expert in horizontal vio-
lence as well as suggestions about style and mechanics.
[Type of Feedback Requested]

As it's a newsletter piece, it'll only take you a few
minutes to read. I can send you an attachment of the
manuscript immediately. It would be helpful to get your
feedback in a week. [Turnaround Time]

If you agree, you'll be acknowledged as a peer editor
in the published article. [Reward]

Please do let me know if this time frame works for you.

As ever, gratefully yours, [Closing]

Kathy
```

This request letter includes the conditions for our agreement: the type of publication project, the desired feedback, the deadline, and the reward. Being as specific as possible about what you're asking of a peer editor when you make your request increases the chances that you'll get the type of peer editing assistance you're seeking.

After you line up your peer editor(s), the next step is to send everything needed to peer edit your work. In my case, I sent Christina the following Publication Worksheet.

Publication Worksheet

My Name: Kathy Heinrich   **My Product:** Newsletter Article

My Idea: Joy Stealing Games

      Topic: What School Nurses Can Do to Stop the Game-Playing

      Focus: Ten steps in stopping joy-stealing games

Purpose: To give back to school nurse group by sharing lessons they taught me about 10 steps in stopping joy-stealing.

Readers: School Nurses

(continues)

Publication Worksheet

Desired Reader Response: To inform and activate them to stop joy-stealing games

Venue/Vehicle: Newsletter

Slant: What Connecticut school nurses taught me about stopping joy-stealing.

One-Sentence Description: This newsletter article describes what I learned from school nurses about helping them stop the joy-stealing games.

As you read through the manuscript, see how closely it follows the Publication Worksheet.

Manuscript

Joy Stealing: What Connecticut School Nurses Taught Me About Stopping the Game-Playing

K.T. Heinrich RN, PhD

Write about a situation with a student, teacher, administrator or parent that's stealing your joy. This article describes what I learned when I asked the 117 school nurses attending your October dinner meeting to respond to this question.

What Is Joy-Stealing?

Joy-stealing games are experiences that rob nurses of their zest, clarity, productivity, feelings of worth, and desire for more connection (Heinrich, 2006). Four roles are played in joy-stealing games: (1) target, (2) joy-stealer, (3) bystander, and (4) ally. From the 117 stories you left with me, it's clear that school nurses play all four roles with students, teachers, secretaries, counselors, administrators, and parents.

(continues)

How One School Nurse Became Her Own Ally

In one of your stories, a school nurse plays the target and a teacher plays the joy-stealer:

> A science teacher wanted a student's abrasions treated "her way." I felt it wasn't medically indicated. She called on the phone yelling, "I told you I wanted them covered." Again, I said it was not medically indicated and I explained why. She was angry when she hung up but she's never done that again.

By staying calm and explaining her rationale from a medical perspective, in language a science teacher could appreciate, this nurse made her point *and* stopped the game.

Ten Steps to Becoming Your Own Ally

1. Recognize when a situation drains your joy.
2. Take a time out! Write down your story.
3. Identify your role. Are you a target, a joy-stealer, a bystander, or an ally?
4. Reach out to your circle of allies, school nurse colleagues, supervisors, principals, etc.
5. Whine, if you feel the need, to your allies.
6. Strategize ways to deal with the situation.
7. Reframe nice. Have the courage and creativity to stand up for what you believe (Koval & Thaler, 2006).
8. Review your "Nice-Person Bill of Rights" (Hiltabiddle & Edelman, 2006).
      Speak up
      Set boundaries
      Take risks
      Value your time
      Be accountable
9. Practice. Allies can help you role-play how to say what you want to say.
10. Move into action. If one strategy doesn't work, try another.

Conclusion

Become an ally to yourself! Then you'll play your part in fostering a zestful school environment with zero-tolerance for joy-stealing games.

References

Heinrich, K. T. (2006, Second Quarter). Joy-stealing games. *Reflections on Nursing Leadership*. Available at: http://www.nursingsociety.org.

Hiltabiddle, T., & Edelman, R. (2006, October 16). In M. Gardner, At Work, 'Nice' Is On The Rise. *The Christian Science Monitor*, 13–14.

Thaler, R., & Koval, L. K. (2006). *The Power of Nice: How to Conquer the Business World with Kindness*. New York: Doubleday.

As you can see, the Worksheet's slant became the manuscript title, and the Worksheet's one-sentence description became the sentence in the manuscript that told readers what to expect from reading this article.

Now imagine yourself in Christina's position by reviewing the worksheet and manuscript from the perspective of a peer editor. Knowing that this manuscript is being submitted to a newsletter tips you off to the *form* as well as the *function* of this manuscript. As far as *form*, newsletter articles are short and written in an informed-conversational writing style in the first person. Readers should be able to scan the headings and know what a newsletter article is about without reading it; reference lists are kept to a minimum—between one and three citations. As for *function*, newsletter articles are informational and devoted to timely topics of interest to the readers who, in this case, are school nurses.

As you can see from her response, Christina's approach to peer editing is to review manuscripts from the reader's point of view, to mirror back what she's learned as a reader, and to ask questions.

Christina's Response

Dear Kathy: ╱**Takes Reader's Point of View**

I've reviewed your joy-stealing manuscript. . .*as a reader* this is what I learned from it . . . By becoming an ally to myself, I can stop the game of joy-stealing. The 10 steps to becoming my own ally are all doable and I can imagine engaging in every step... Thank you, I will use these strategies with my nurses.

                                    ╱**Mirror Back What I Learned**

In the story, the school nurse started as a target and ended as her own ally through the strategies of staying calm and explaining her rationale. Beautiful! If she can become her own ally, so can I. It also gives hope to those of us who may start as the joy-stealer or bystander.

                                    ╱**Clarifying Question**

This is what I wondered about... I wanted a little more. I am a bit confused about how I can stop the game playing by being my own ally when being an ally is one of the four roles played in joy-stealing games.

Christina

Christina's feedback both confirms that readers will get the message that I'm trying to convey and offers a suggestion for revision. The following is the e-mail message that I sent in response to Christina's feedback.

Reply

Dear Christina:

Wow, you're a wonderfully fast reader!!!

Thanks for your close reading. It's gratifying to know that you, as my reader, picked up the messages meant to be conveyed. I will take your "wanting more" into account as I revise—the editor said it has to be 400 words so I have to be a bit clipped :)

Happy day,

Kathy

Note that I addressed Christina's editorial question directly to acknowledge her feedback. I made the following change to the conclusion of the final manuscript based on Christina's feedback.

Change Made

Conclusion

~~Become an ally to yourself.~~ *To be an ally for someone else, you must first be an ally to yourself.* Then you can play a part in fostering a zestful school environment with zero-tolerance for joy-stealing games.

Once an article is published, I like to close the circle of generosity by sending peer editors a formal letter of thanks along with a copy of publications with the acknowledgment where their name appears. In this instance, when I went to snail mail the article to Christina I noticed that the acknowledgment was missing. When I followed up with the editor, I learned that the final draft had not included the acknowledgment so it was not published. In my follow-up communication, I explained and apologized to Christina for this oversight.

No matter what happens, peer editing is a relationship between author and peer editor, and it's important to request, respond to, and reward your colleague's generosity accordingly.

TIP

Request and acknowledge colleagues' generosity for peer editing your work.

What to Do When Receiving or Giving Peer Editing Feedback

73

At times I have to pull back and remind myself of how the manuscript exists in the life of the writer and know how exquisitely sensitive the writer is going to be to rejection or critical comment, and I try to make an extra effort to read the work with an open and attentive mind.

C. Michael Curtis

If writing takes courage, having one's writing peer edited is just as courageous. Depending on your experiences with peer editors, some of you might even call it suicidal. I'll never forget what happened during the first class of a course when I explained that students would peer edit each other's papers. One student raised her hand and asked if this was a requirement to pass the course. She almost came to tears recalling how she'd been "crucified" by a fellow student's feedback on a writing assignment. Her story made my heart hurt and reinforced why a structured approach for peer editing is so crucial.

It's often difficult for nurses to give each other feedback, we either kill with kindness or kill off with criticism. Because there's no script for peer editing, this chapter outlines three tasks for writers and peer editors that bring balance to their critiques. Up until now, we've been talking about peer-editing relationships that involve an electronic exchange. The following principles apply to peer-editing sessions conducted face-to-face to ensure that they are productive and respectful experiences for both parties.

When in the role of the writer:

1. **Take responsibility for getting feedback that you want.** Peer editing becomes safer when authors, not peer editors, hold the reins. In addition to specifying whether they want expert, general audience, or stylistic feedback, authors need to ask for the type of feedback they are seeking. Remember the mathematical shorthand for peer-mentoring feedback: only positive (+); only what needs to be fixed (–); or positive and what needs to be fixed (+/–; see Chapter 44). It's the same for peer editing. Whether authors ask for positives or not, I offer positives first, because appreciation frees them up to listen to what might need to be changed.

2. **Listen silently to all feedback.** When you're the author, it's easy to get into apologizing or making excuses for your writing. Don't! Stay silent when your peer editor is offering feedback. Soak in the comments. A good way to avoid the temptation to defend or deflect is to take notes on your peer editor's feedback. Then, after your peer editor finishes speaking, ask questions to clarify your understanding of feedback given.

3. **Decide which feedback to follow or to ignore later.** As the author, take responsibility for what you write. Make only those changes that make sense to you given your readership and the nature of your vehicle. By being the decision maker, you remain true to yourself and to your work. The downside is that there's no one else to blame when your manuscripts are rejected.

Switching to the role of peer editor, clarity and kindness are the by-words. C. Michael Curtis puts it well when he speaks of being sensitive to "how the manuscript exists in the life of the writer."[1] Keep in mind that people are as apprehensive about sharing their writing as they are about talking about sex or finances.

When in the role of peer editor:

1. **Respond to the writing, not the writer.** In this case, the peer-editing relationship involves three entities: the author, the peer editor, and the work. Focus on the *work* when giving your feedback. For example, instead of saying "you" and "here you say," speak about "this piece" and "in this paragraph, it says."

2. **Use "I" messages.** When peer editing another's writing, speak from the reader's perspective: "For me, as the reader, this term is new. A definition would help me understand."

3. **Be as specific as possible in your feedback.** Comments such as "unclear what you mean here" don't help the author. It's much more helpful to say, "I am unclear about the meaning of this sentence. There's two good ideas in it. Unbundle them and write a sentence devoted to each idea." You may even want to tell the author what the two ideas are. Leave it up to the author to figure out how to fix it.

In sum, as the one receiving peer editing, listen. As the one giving peer editing, be as sensitive as you are candid. So, whether you're the author or the peer editor, the key is to treat the other person as you would want to be treated.

TIP

Peer editing is a relationship for which both the writer and the editor bear responsibility.

Reference

1. Miller, L. (2000, September). An interview with C. Michael Curtis. *The Writer's Chronicle, 33*(1), 43–44.

How to
Peer Edit

Imagination is more important than knowledge.

Albert Einstein

How do you nurture the voice of writers? C. Michael Curtis' response is an inspiration for peer editors:

> Among other things by not squashing it. That is, by letting writers use whatever voice they like while holding them accountable to the wish for clarity and coherence that any serious reader demands. I wouldn't insist that a writer do things the way I do them or the way I most admire. I would want to leave open the possibility of literary achievement that is unexpected, idiosyncratic. I'm always torn between a desire to encourage the kind of work I most admire and a desire to honor what is particular to the work of the student.[1]

Honoring what is particular to the work of writers while holding them accountable for the clarity and coherence due their readers—this is the art of peer editing. Put another way, peer editing is *not* rewriting. Peer editing is the skillful giving of feedback in a way that allows authors to see their writing through the eyes of an attentive reader.

Now that you've read about enacting the roles of peer edited and peer editor, this chapter introduces a simple and effective way to peer edit. As nonthreatening as it is insight-provoking for the author, we'll walk through each step of this three-step approach together. The following is an excerpt from a student journal entry written in response to a class on the art of giving feedback. First, read through this student's entry with "beginner's mind" to gain an appreciation for what is being said.

> I really enjoyed today's class. Elaine is a wonderful speaker. Sharing feedback is always a topic that needs attention, especially in an interactive class. Many people do not know how to give constructive, positive feedback. I think people mix up constructive feedback with negative feedback. What I mean is that when people give feedback they think constructive feedback is better approached with the negative aspects of the subject being evaluated. When you begin with a negative comment, it is often difficult to repair the damage.
>
> When I sat down to share my drawing of autumn with another student in class, I definitely felt uncomfortable and the first thing out of her mouth was why do you have flowers in a fall scene? Of course, I got defensive and was really put off with anything further that she had to say. I like flowers and we were told to draw our vision of fall and for me that includes flowers. When we were asked again to give the other person feedback on how they could change their drawing of fall, she continued to focus on those darn flowers even after I explained why I put them in there and the experience was not positive.
>
> I will say that her sentence on how I could change my interpretation of fall was improved after her initial feedback. I just wish she could of said something positive about my drawing, I already felt terrible because I cannot draw.
>
> I follow the steps Elaine gave us in class when I precept new nurses, and the experience is definitely more positive for all. Feedback should be clear, start with a positive, focus on the behavior, offer alternatives, use "I" statements and be aware of the tone of your voice.

How was that for you? Were you tempted to correct rather than read? For me, it's always difficult to read for comprehension, because I'm so used to grabbing my pen to correct errors in spelling and grammar. Drop that pen!

After reading the excerpt a second time, free-write a mirroring statement; that is, tell the writer what you understand about what you're reading.

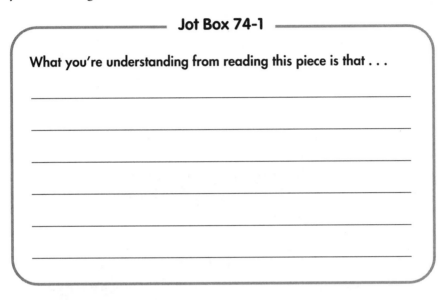

Jot Box 74-1

What you're understanding from reading this piece is that . . .

_____

_____

_____

_____

_____

_____

What was that like for you? In the beginning, I found myself feeling afraid that I wouldn't know what the writer was saying. That may be because I'm already thinking ahead to how to improve on what's been said. I've included my free-write so you can see another example of a mirroring response.

What I'm understanding from reading this is that . . . you were learning the principles for giving feedback in this class and during the practice session, you experienced an interaction with a classmate that hurt your feelings and violated the principle of starting feedback off with a positive.

Mirroring allows authors to see their writing through the reader's eyes and three questions show where assumptions or lack of clarity might leave readers confused (see Jot Box 74-2).

Now read this excerpt a final time and formulate three questions that begin with the phrase, "As a reader, I'd like to know more about . . ."

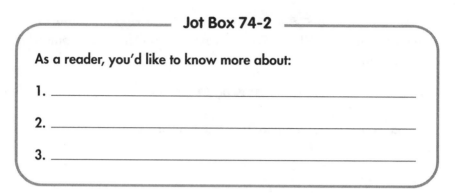

============ **Jot Box 74-2** ============

As a reader, you'd like to know more about:

1. _____

2. _____

3. _____

How was it for you to peer edit another's writing by reading through, free-writing a mirroring response, and then asking questions? Can you see how your three questions might open this author to insights about what needs to be changed and how to make changes? Here are my three questions.

As a reader, I'd like to know more about:

1. What were the reasons that you found Elaine such a wonderful speaker?
2. Why is it "especially important" to discuss feedback-giving in interactive classrooms?
3. Given your response to your partner's criticism of your flowers, do you want to add a sentence about being sensitive to another's feelings when giving feedback?

The genius of this three-step approach is that it establishes trust and leaves writers in charge of editing their own work. By using this combination of reading, mirroring, and questioning, you leave it to authors to respond as they see fit. Notice how this simple approach keeps your feedback focused on the writing, stated in the first person "I," and specific.

TIP

When you're asked to be a peer editor, read, mirror, and question.

References

1. Miller, L. (2000, September). An interview with C. Michael Curtis. *The Writer's Chronicle, 33*(1), 43–44.

How to Celebrate Revisions and Thrive on Rejections

75

There is no such thing as great writers, there are only great rewriters.

Noah Lukeman

Penelope submitted a manuscript to a refereed, nursing journal before she read *Dare to Share*. Why did the editor return Penelope's manuscript without even sending it out to his external reviewers? It turns out that Penelope submitted an "A" paper she'd written as a student without revising it for his journal. Penelope is not alone. According to Suzanne Hall Johnson, the "school-paper rejection" is the most common reason for editors returning manuscripts.[1]

To make sure that this doesn't happen to you, revise papers, theses, and dissertations so that your manuscript:

- States the main idea in the introduction, rather than waiting until the end.
- Includes only the content appropriate to the level of the readers.
- Uses references selectively to support, rather than to validate, ideas.

Now back to Penelope. After reading *Dare to Share*, she filled out a Publication Worksheet; queried an editor who expressed interest; asked an expert, a general reader, and a style peer editor to review her manuscript;

and followed the author guidelines. She submitted her manuscript a month ago and hasn't heard back. This isn't unusual. Although editors often respond to queries within 24 to 72 hours, the typical turnaround on reviewing manuscripts can be anywhere from a month to a year, with the median being four to six months.

Penelope's story might play out in two different ways, the ending is up to her.

Scenario 1: Revision

Penelope gets a letter from the editor saying he'll be happy to review her manuscript after she revises it using the enclosed reviewers' comments as a guide. After all she did to prepare her manuscript for this particular journal, Penelope is ready to forget about getting published. She doesn't know how close his request for revision is to an acceptance. When authors make the recommended changes, their manuscripts are almost always published. That's why Marilyn Oermann says, "If you're asked to revise your manuscript, DO IT ASAP and include an item-by-item response to comments from reviewers." When you get your next request for revision, don't forget to use your judgment as an author. When a reviewer's comment doesn't make sense, don't make the revision. Do offer your rationale for not making the suggested change in your item-by-item response to the editor. Making a reasoned case can often persuade an editor to honor your decision. Even though I often resent making revisions in the moment, I have learned that they can be blessings in disguise. The revision is always better than the original version.

Let's replay this scenario with Penelope receiving a rejection letter.

Scenario 2: Rejection

Penelope receives a letter from an editor that says thanks but no thanks. While nurse-authors' responses to manuscript rejection may range from disappointed to devastated, Penelope's feelings are closer to devastation. There's no question that rejections are hard to take, no matter who you are, how much you've written, or how confident you are that your manuscript is worthy of publication. That said, Suzanne Hall Johnson brings a fresh perspective when she says, "Don't be afraid of rejection. If that happens, most editors will give you advice on how to revise." She's right. In the case of nonrefereed periodicals, most editors explain their reasons for rejection. And in the case of refereed periodicals, editors often send along the actual feedback from the external reviewers. Marilyn Oermann offers the practical steps to take, "If your paper is rejected, revise it using the reviewer comments, reformat it, and send to the next journal on your original list. Keep sending until your manuscript is published." Published authors aren't necessarily the best writers, we're the ones willing to persevere through revisions and rejections. I've gotten so many manuscripts rejected that I've got my response down to a science. After ripping open an editor's letter and reading the opening phrase, "We're sorry to inform you . . . ," I throw the letter on the floor and leave it there for a few days. When I've calmed down enough, I reread the letter and use the editors' or reviewers' suggestions to make revisions. Where else can you get free editorial advice tailored to your manuscript?

So now that Penelope's situation allowed us to play out both scenarios, I hope that when those requests for revisions or rejections come in, as they will, you'll take a page from our editors to:

- Send manuscripts in expecting you'll have to revise and being joyous when you don't have to.
- Be unafraid of rejection. When it happens, most editors will give you advice on how to revise.
- Take a revision request or a rejection as an opportunity to press forward.

It may be too much to expect you to actually celebrate revisions and thrive on rejections, but learning to roll with them is all part of getting published.

TIP
When you persevere, you'll be proud of the published product that revisions make possible.

Reference

1. Johnson, S. H. (1991, Summer). Avoiding the "school paper style" rejection. *Nurse Author & Editor: A Newsletter for Nurse Authors, Editors and Editorial Review Boards, 1*(3), 130–135.

How to Work Smart by Turning Co-Presenters into Co-Authors

76

Perceive all conflict as patterns of energy seeking harmonious balance as elements in a whole.

Dhyani Ywahoo

Let's say that your presentation was so well-received that you and your co-presenter want to turn it into a publication. You assume that dividing up your writing project the way you divided your presentation will work just fine. When you meet after you've each written your section of the presentation, you realize that pulling together a manuscript isn't going to be so easy. It's clear that someone will have to translate your separate sections into a piece that reads like one author wrote it. That's when your co-presenter says she wants to be "first author" because she's coming up for a promotion. Because she's a less experienced writer, this unifying task will fall to you. You resent the idea of doing that amount of work without your name being listed as the first author, but you're hesitant to say this to her because it sounds selfish. You begin to wonder if your relationship will survive this publication.

There's a better way. Let's replay this scenario using a work-smart approach. When you work smart, projects are divided into two phases: a presentation phase and a publication phase:

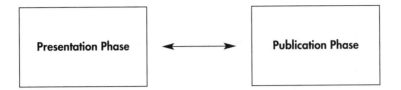

FIGURE 76-1   Two Phases of Work-Smart Projects

In this sequence, an invitation to present becomes an invitation to publish. Asking the work-smart question—*Do we want to turn our presentation into a publication?*—prior to the presentation, following the presentation, and before the publication phase keeps this possibility open throughout the project (see Table 76-1).

TABLE 76-1   Work-Smart Tasks During Presentation and Publication Phases

Pose Work-Smart Question	Phases in Project
Invitation	Pre-Presentation Session
	Presentation
Exploration	Post-Presentation Session
Negotiation	Pre-Publication Session

Invitation During Pre-Presentation Session

Do we want to turn our presentation into a publication? Discussing publishing possibilities prior to initiating presentation projects keeps both phases of work-smart projects in sight throughout. With two products to consider, your decision making about roles and responsibilities related to presenting and publishing projects becomes easier. This way, before you even agree to co-present, you discuss issues like whose name will be listed first on the presentation and on the publication. As you complete your Presentation Worksheet, you're keeping your Publication Worksheet in mind. In conducting your literature search, you're a presenter in search of the latest ideas to share as well as an author seeking a venue. As you review audience-participants' evaluations, you're already considering how to use their feedback to refine your publication.

Exploration During the Post-Presentation Session

Do we want to turn our presentation into a publication? After bringing the presenting phase to closure by reviewing the "What Worked and Future Changes" worksheet and participant evaluations, you're ready to revisit the work-smart question. Should you and your co-presenters agree that you want to explore a co-authorship collaboration, set a time for a negotiation session that takes place before the publication process. Prior to this session, answer the following three questions on your own:

1. What do I want from my involvement in this writing project?
2. What can I contribute to this writing project?
3. What's worked well with the authoring or co-authoring arrangements in my past?

Negotiation During Pre-Publication Session

Do we want to turn our presentation into a publication? Sharing your responses to the three questions you prepared before this session sets the stage for negotiating the nature and conditions of your collaboration during the publication phase. Depending on what's discussed, you may decide (1) that the project ends with the presentation; (2) that your participation ends with the presentation phase; or (3) that you want to proceed with the publication phase. Should you agree to collaborate on a publication, a new contract and covenant are negotiated. As you may remember from Section II, contracts are agreements that deal with the details of the project like delineating perks and responsibilities (see Chapter 34). Your contract specifies the following:

- The roles and responsibilities of each collaborator (e.g., co-author, peer editor, etc.)
- The order in which the authors' names appear
- The time frame for the project, including deadlines.

Covenants, as in the case of presentations, attend to the relational dimensions of your writing collaboration.

Like all relationships, creative collaborations require mindful communication to keep them zestful and on task.[1,2] By asking the work-smart question, assumptions such as the ones you and your co-presenter made in our hypothetical example that opened the chapter are replaced by reflection and dialogue. Collaborators who keep asking each other this one question are more likely to emerge from projects with colleague–friendships so vibrant that they'll seek out future opportunities for collaboration.

TIP

Ask the work-smart question to transition from presentation to publication projects with mindfulness.

References

1. Heinrich, K. T. (1997, Spring). Is your co-author relationship on the rocks?: How to know and what to do. *Nurse Author & Editor: A Newsletter for Nurse Authors, Editors, and Editorial Board Members, 7*(2), 4, 7–8.
2. Heinrich, K. T. (1995, Fall). Co-authorship: Turning pitfalls into pleasures. *Nurse Author & Editor: A Newsletter for Nurse Authors, Editors, and Editorial Board Members, 5*(4), 1–3.

How a Nurse-Author's Story May Change Your Life

77

You can think of balancing your life in two ways: One I call both/and, while the other is either/or. A lot of people think they can either go the professional route or choose to be a wife and mother. I like the both/and approach. You can have both and do both. You can enjoy a family life while leading a professional life. I really believe I am one of those people who had it all.

Shirley Sears Chater

As I was writing the chapters in this section, I wondered how to show you what it's really like to be a nurse-author. All of it, from the highs of inspiration and getting a thumbs up from an editor to those times when even the most eye-glittering idea has lost its sparkle and the words just won't come. The answer appeared, quite literally, during lunch. As we spoke about *Dare to Share* over salads and iced teas, my colleague–friend Laurel Halloran said, "I hope you're telling your readers the how-to's. That's what I always wondered about before I got published, how do nurses go about the actual writing process." After stammering something about publication worksheets and timelines, inspiration hit and I asked Laurel to share her "how-tos" with you.

When she agreed without a moment's hesitation, I almost hugged her. After reading what she has to say, you'll feel like hugging her too. Her chapter offers a rare glimpse into the life of a nurse-author. Laurel's down-to-earth sense of humor and practical suggestions sum up the steps she takes in writing her monthly column for a practitioner journal. She shares everything from her filing system to her creative timeout strategies, not to mention how she juggles being a writer and a mom, a wife, a practicing N.P., and a full-time faculty member.

You'll get a chuckle out of her bait-and-switch tactic where she pretends to wash the dinner dishes as a way to clear the kitchen of family members so she can steal a few hours between after-dinner and bed-time for writing. She's even honest about how she perseveres when she doesn't feel like writing or isn't sure that she can write. And how, in spite of it all, she manages to get her manuscripts to her editors on time, every time.

Laurel is the best kind of nurse-author, one of the ones who loves to mentor other authors as much as she loves to read[1] and to write. So, if you're worried that you really don't get what this writing thing is all about, don't wait another minute. Read Laurel's chapter to see how she pulls together all the steps and strategies shared in this section. You'll come away with a much better idea of how to work writing into your busy life.

Reference

1. Prose, F. (2006). *Reading like a writer: A guide for people who love books and those who want to write them.* New York: HarperCollins.

How My Students Helped Me to Actualize a Childhood Dream

78

Laurel Halloran, PhD, APRN

Sit down and put everything down that comes into your head and then you're a writer. But an author is one who can judge his own stuff's worth, without pity, and destroy most of it.

Colette

I am a nurse practitioner, a mom, a wife, and an educator. I'm also an author. And here I'm going to make a confession: I am not brilliant. This would not surprise any of my friends and family, but it might surprise those who have been reading columns that I have written for *Advance for Nurse Practitioners* for the past two years. Although I have always had an interest in writing, I came to it late in my career. I was one of those kids who vacillated between getting a liberal arts degree in English and becoming a nurse. My father—interested in my being self-supporting—encouraged nursing. It has been a wonderful career, but I always knew something was missing. I wanted to write. Submitting a few things early on in my career, I was unsuccessful in getting published. Then I gave up for a while. I found it much easier to present than to publish and, fortunately for me, they were deemed equal in terms of promotion and tenure at the university where I teach. I wanted to write, I was just scared. And I didn't really know how to go about it which may be why I always want to know *how* successful authors go about getting published.

That's, in fact, where the idea for this chapter came from. Kathy and I went through our doctoral program together. We even had the same major advisor—now there's a bonding experience! We try to meet with some regularity just to catch up on each other's lives. As we talked about this book, I said that I hoped *Dare to Share* included a "how to do it" chapter. She asked me to write the chapter, so here we are. What a great lunch!

I swear that I had not seen Kathy's chapters prior to sitting down to put my thoughts on paper. I found it interesting that my process for writing is very similar to the structure described in Chapters 58 to 70 (Section III). This chapter shows you how I go about creating something that others want to read, because I want you to know that you can do this, too. The fact that you're reading this book may mean that there's an author inside of you waiting to be unleashed. If this thought resonates with something deep within, you'll know what I say is true.

Inspiration from Consternation

My writing for *Advance for Nurse Practitioners* came straight from my distress over the "file-drawer syndrome" (**slant**). As an educator, I was watching too many master's students file their theses in a drawer after graduation without ever taking their research findings "on the road" (**eye-glittering idea**). So, one day when I was noodling around on the computer, I created four word files and titled them—"writing an abstract," "doing a poster presentation," "doing a podium presentation," "writing a manuscript"—then I shut off the computer and walked the dog.

Over the next few weeks, I added to each file bit by bit. Once I had a file pretty much completed, I would put it away for a few days. Then I would go back over it with fresh eyes and edit, remembering to use both spell check and grammar check. When I gave them to the students to read, one said to me "this makes it look possible." AH HA! If my students liked them, maybe others would also. But who (**audience**)? Many graduate programs, including ours, require master's students to do a "research- or project-based thesis." What journals do such students read in their off time? I didn't really know, so as a practicing nurse practitioner

I picked one that I read, which is how I came to pitch the idea of a series of four articles to *Advance for Nurse Practitioners.*[1–4] I'd say the rest is history except that I'm only getting started.

I owe a lot of my success in writing to two groups of people. If this sounds like the start of an Academy Award speech, I promise I'll be brief! The first group is the students who encouraged me to put myself out there and submit my manuscripts for publication. Not only did students tell me the manuscripts were good, they helped me to evaluate which journals would be appropriate and celebrated my success along with me. The second group is the fantastic editors with whom I work at *Advance for Nurse Practitioners.* They encourage me, provide sound advice, tell me when I'm off the mark without making me want to open a bottle of wine, and have become friends. Because writing can be a lonely business, you need editors like them who say "I think you have something here—please keep working on it" (**support circle**).

How I Go About Writing About What I Do

Step 1: Where to Start

I think anyone who writes also likes to read. Many times I'll pick up a journal, cut out an article of particular interest and place it in a topic-labeled, file folder. I use these articles to update lectures or to provide references and documentation for manuscripts. One caveat is to keep your file updated by tossing outdated articles. If you don't, you'll end up sitting down to write your article on lung cancer and find articles from 1995 in your folder. The general rule is no readings older than five years, unless it's a classic.

When you search the literature, put a time limit on how long you collect resources so as not to lose your ideas in and amongst those in the literature. It's rare to find the perfect article or book that pulls it all together. That's good news! I know Pam Walker stressed this in her chapter on literature searches (Chapter 27, Section II), but it's so important, I'll say it again. The best place to find your unique slant is to look for what hasn't been written about your topic.

One activity with no term limit is collecting quotations. When I read or hear a quote that resonates, I jot it down in a small *Dare to Share* notebook that I carry for just such a purpose. I bought mine at Kate's

Paperie in New York City; they have a Web site, too. Just the other day I was listening to a friend, who had had a difficult time conceiving, talk about her new baby and her success at work. When I asked her how she manages both, she said to me "Sometimes when you can achieve one of your dreams you start to believe that all the others are possible." Isn't that beautiful? I wrote this quotation into my notebook because I'll definitely find a place for it somewhere.

I also read books on writing. If you want to write, reading is the best teacher. My favorites are *The Artist's Way* by Julia Cameron,[5] or really anything written by Julia Cameron, and *On Writing* by Stephen King.[6] I never read Stephen King books. Frankly, I still think that "Misery" was the scariest movie I've ever seen. His book on writing is a jewel.

Step 2: Right Place, Time, Priority, and Voice

Ideas for columns come from a list of approved topics that are mutually generated and agreed upon. To get the ball rolling for my next *Advance* column, I start by sending a list of ideas to my editors who may add or delete ideas. If I'm having difficulty with a topic, I'll ask if I can make a substitution or get their input on approaching the topic. The columns have submission deadlines attached. Once I've settled on a topic, I give myself a deadline, written in stone, as to when the first draft must be completed. It's usually at least a week before the column is due—I'm Irish, and we're very superstitious—I want to be ready for everything from a virus to a computer meltdown.

As I said before, I keep files on topics of interest. When I'm writing about a specific topic, I pull out the file and briefly review the current materials (10 minutes). This is something that I might do when I am waiting in a doctor's office or for the car's oil to be changed—or just catching a cup of coffee at the local Starbucks. I jot down ideas and outlines if they come to me. Then I sit down to write.

After dinner is usually a quiet time in my house. I make like I'm washing dishes, everyone disappears, and I have a couple of hours free to write (**time**). My retreat is a small office set up with my computer and Internet access in a spare bedroom (**place**). Once there, I sit my butt in the chair (**priority**). This is usually the most difficult part of the writing process for me. I can think of 20 other things I should/could be doing. If I start to itch to do the laundry, I stop and read one of the inspirational quotes taped on the doors of the armoire that houses my computer table. My current favorite is one that says:

> The essential question is not "How busy are you?" but "What are you busy at?" Are you doing what fulfills you? Someday is not an eighth day of the week. I hope this encourages you to claim time for the passions that make you love your life.
>
> —Anonymous

When I'm having trouble getting started, reading this gets me going **(still-point strategy)**. Once in that receptive-creative mode, I put the dirty laundry on hold as I sit down again. A famous author once said "I write when inspiration hits me . . . and I make sure it hits me at 9 A.M. every morning." There will never be a perfect time to write. Kids will need to be driven somewhere, lectures will need to be done, patients will want to be seen, and the dog will throw up. Don't wait for a time when it will be easier. Sit down to write. As T. S. Elliot wrote, "One starts an action simply because one must do something."

I also find that if I commit to a 5- to 10-minute writing session I usually last much longer. When I start to write, I literally put down every thought I have in my head on the paper with no thoughts about editing or correct spelling **(free-write)**. You tend to lose your creative momentum if you get caught up in whether the appropriate word is "which" or "that." That's why God invented spell and grammar check. As long as you remember to do it before you send it out, you're fine. Once I'm done for the night I save the file, e-mail it to myself (see, I am superstitious), and forget about it.

The next day or so I go on with my usual routine. Often I'll print out a hard copy and just read through it. Then I walk the dog and use the quiet time to just think about whether this says what I want it to say **(voice)**. I get some of my best ideas while walking. There must be some connection between exercise and brain activity. I might revise again at this point—and remember, I still have some time before my deadline. More likely, I'll go back in and spell and grammar check. Because my columns have a word limit, I also use word count. I don't get it down to the exact number of words I need, but I get it close. This saves the editor from having to do a lot of additional work. Then I go through it from the beginning to see if I'm hitting the target of what I really wanted to say (**know-how**). I make sure that I integrate some personal experiences. After that, I spell check and grammar check again (**perfectionism**) and save the file as revised. My final step is sending off the attachment to my editor by e-mail with a personal note a good two days before its due date.

Step 3: Impostor Feelings

I've been writing this column for two years, and I have another secret to share. Until I get an e-mail back from my editor that she thinks it's okay, I doubt whether I can write at all. Joanie Chestnut from high school was right when she told me that my writing was "trite." Now who uses a word like that in high school? I thought that it was only me who thought this way; I was even getting used to the crazy looks I got from colleagues when I mentioned my angst, but I found that I'm not alone. The Imposter Syndrome is real! Julia Cameron, who has published over 20 books, as well as musicals, screenplays, and poetry, writes, "I've gotten used to the two horsemen of a writing career: the desire to write and the fear that this time I won't be able to pull it off."[5]

When not worrying about my writing, I worry that I've attached the file incorrectly or that I've attached the wrong file. I actually did do this once and sent a major nursing journal a file that had not even been spell checked. The reality is that submitting something for publication is scary. I can't take away your worries. What I can tell you is that the rewards *far* outweigh the risks. The most famous of authors—think Hemingway—have had lots of misses.

Step 4: A Shift in Attitude, a Gain in Gratitude

This step should really be titled "Leave your ego at the door" or "Learn by your mistakes." Editors make changes to manuscripts. Well versed in what their readers want, they are experts in keeping the essence of a manuscript while fitting it into those pages in the journal. Trust your editors. Tell them you trust them. Thank them for doing their jobs. Let me tell you what can happen when you don't. I sent off a manuscript to a certain journal and the editors agreed to rereview it *if* I made suggested changes. Instead of making the changes they suggested, I stuck to my guns and only made some changes. The manuscript was politely and very quickly declined. In retrospect, I messed up on one of the basics. I sent a manuscript written in a formal academic, "research-y" style to a journal with an informed-conversational style. Not a match. I'm in the process of revising it once again in hopes of finding a vehicle with an audience that reads the research stuff I'm so passionate about.

Lesson learned. As an author, you've got a decision to make. Either choose a vehicle that fits your manuscript or fit your manuscript to a vehicle. When you treat editors as collaborators and search for the best home for your manuscripts, you'll have more opportunities to publish and we'll get the chance to read your work.

Final Thoughts

This chapter shared the small steps, strategies, and skills that I've found most useful in my writing process. Yes, I'm lucky to have found a voice, a journal, editors, and readers who enjoy what I have to say. But remember that I was 50 years old before I had the courage to put myself out there. Can you write about what you do everyday? The only way to find out is to take the dare to share. No matter what your age, if writing is calling to you, here's a question to help you make the decision. Do you want to be a year older and writing about what you do? Or do you just want to be a year older?

If writing is your dream, don't wait another minute. Pin this quote from Jean Claude Monet written when he was 85 years young on your armoire door, sit your butt down, and start writing.

> The further I go, the more I understand that it is imperative to work a great deal to achieve what I seek. More than ever, I am easily disgusted in things that come in a single stroke. In the end, I am excited by the need to render what I feel. I vow to live on not unproductively . . . because it seems to me, that I will make progress.

TIP

Reach out to allies along the way whether they're your patients, students, teachers, colleague–friends, or editors.

References

1. Halloran, L. (2006, January). Writing for publication. *Advance for Nurse Practitioners, 14*(1), 75.
2. Halloran, L. (2005, December). Poise at the podium. *Advance for Nurse Practitioners, 13*(12), 66.
3. Halloran, L. (2005, November). Picture pages. *Advance for Nurse Practitioners, 13*(11), 67.
4. Halloran, L. (2005, October). Abstract reasoning. *Advance for Nurse Practitioners, 13*(10), 84.
5. Cameron, J. (1992). *The artist's way: A spiritual path to higher creativity.* New York: Putnam.
6. King, S. (2000). *On writing: A memoir of the craft.* New York: Scribner.

Conclusion: Commit to Writing About What You Do

79

We write to taste life twice, in the moment and in retrospection.

Anais Nin

When Laurel sent me a card with the saying above on the cover, it seemed the perfect way to close. Having completed this section, you've learned how to taste life three times—live an experience, present it, and write about it. With this in mind, let's find out how your three nurse companions responded to the question, "Where are you with working smart by turning a presentation into a publication?"

Keri wrote:

> I got so excited after reading Laurel's chapter, I felt like I knew her! Her informed-conversational writer's voice is the one I'd like to use in publishing my presentation ideas. I've written a query letter to her editors at *Advance for Nurse Practitioners* to see if they are interested in reviewing my manuscript combining reflections on my first year in practice with the findings from my thesis.

Betty's free-write reads:

> When I agreed to turn my Nurse's Day dinner presentation, "We've Got Stories: Let's Help Each Other Share Them,"

into a manuscript for our hospital newsletter, I needn't have worried about the word count. After completing my Publication Worksheet, I tried free-writing, mind-mapping, and outlining my manuscript. Discarding any ideas not related to my slant made it easy to end up with a manuscript well within the 750-word limit. The newsletter editor is thrilled with it, and he's publishing it in the next issue. I can't say enough about how supportive he was during this whole process. I'm really getting hooked on this work-smart rhythm of present one/publish one.

Justin writes:

This working-smart idea is great! With my instructor's help, I've submitted a poster presentation proposal based on that controversial classroom debate to the NSNA [National Student Nurses' Association] convention conveners. By setting out a timeline with small steps, I can move a project forward, and there's always something to do—no matter how much or how little time I have available. Our next goal for our men's group is to submit a proposal for a paper to be delivered at the regional conference of the "Association of Male Nurses."

As you can see, Keri, Betty, and Justin are tasting life three times by working smart and turning their lived experience into presentations and publications. Before you free-write your own response to the same question as your nurse companions answered (see Jot Box 79-1), refresh your memory by reviewing the 15 Powerful Practices for Working Smart (see Information Box 79-1).

Keeping these practices in mind, it's your turn to answer the same question as did your companions in Jot Box 79-1.

When you commit to writing about what you do, you'll find yourself living life more vibrantly, because every experience becomes a potential opportunity to share what you do by working smart.

TIP
Work smart by turning your presentations into publications.

─── **Information Box 79-1** ───

Powerful Practices for Working Smart: 15 Ways to Transform Presentations into Publications

1. Find ways to make writing easier.
2. Accommodate your writing challenges.
3. Enlist your sweetheart to take on your inner critic.
4. Find your voice.
5. Expand your repertoire of writing styles.
6. Write yourself into still point.
7. Complete a Publication Worksheet.
8. Negotiate mindful collaborations whether contributions involve acknowledgments or co-authorships.
9. Commit to your timeline.
10. Query editors.
11. Reframe requests for revision and rejections as opportunities.
12. Translate your Kolb-It design into an outline.
13. Ask for peer editing and decide what changes to make.
14. Revise, revise, revise.
15. Celebrate your successes.

─── **Jot Box 79-1** ───

Where are you with regard to working smart by turning a presentation into a publication?

_____

_____

_____

_____

_____

Small Steps to Cultivate Support Circles

Introduction: Who Are These Nurses Called Colleague–Friends?

80

*Blessed is the influence of one true,
loving soul upon another.*

George Eliot

Scaring myself silly not long ago brought home the importance of having colleague–friends. At the time I agreed to turn a workshop of mine into an audio-Web seminar, I could barely "do" PowerPoint. Sponsored by the National League for Nursing (NLN), audio-Web seminars enable nurse-educators to sit at their laptops in nursing schools across the country while they listen as the voice of a presenter sitting at her home computer talks them through a PowerPoint slide presentation. Six days before my audio-Web seminar, I found out that my Mac wouldn't interface with the system. Where, at this late date, was I going to get a PC and someone who knew how to work it?

During a restless night, I remembered that two colleagues—Katharine White and Judy Murphy—had asked if they could attend this seminar. These expert PC users lived only an hour away. The next morning I e-mailed a message tagged "A New Partnership Opportunity," asking for their help in exchange for attending. By day's end, Katharine and Judy had cleared their schedules. A week later, buoyed by the warmth and expertise of two of my favorite colleagues, I focused on presenting as Katharine manned the computer and Judy helped field audience questions.

347

Katharine and Judy are the colleague–friends who helped make that audio-Web seminar possible. Barter, trade, it's reciprocal. Katharine or Judy know that when they ask they can count on my help. The idea of mutually beneficial relationships with colleagues may be new to you. Nurses are prone to seeing themselves as helpers and their patients, students and colleagues as recipients of that help. Trade this one-directional view for a "partnership perspective"[1] and you agree to get as much as you give. Ask the following two questions of colleagues—How can I help you? How can you help me?—and your professional life will change.

Then, wherever and whenever you meet colleague–friends, you'll share what's happening in your professional life with a sprinkling of the personal mixed into the conversation. They're the ones you'll ask to help turn proposals into eye-glittering presentations and "shitty first drafts" into splendid publications. As they invite you to explore new opportunities, your confidence will soar as your list of projects, presentations, and publications lengthens. In sum, colleague–friends are the heart, soul, mind, and spirit of support circles.

A support circle can include co-presenters, co-authors, peer mentors, peer editors and partners. All those who care about you *and* dare you to share. When these collegial relationships are mutually beneficial and reciprocal, they're called *partnerships.* To give you a feel for partnership relationships, I've asked some colleague–friends to write the storytelling chapters. An entrepreneur explains how peer mentoring has changed her life, two nurses share what they've learned from spending the last year peer editing *Dare to Share*; and three educators with a shared professional passion describe how their partnership balances competition and connection.

Intertwining show with tell, each of their chapters is followed by a chapter that underscores a relational strategy or skill described in their stories. Reading these chapters may remind you how much of this language of sharing has seeped into your vocabulary. If you didn't before, you'll understand how their partnership relationships with colleague–friends can become a sunny field where they can give free rein to dare-to-share ideas in the company of playmates they trust.

The key to successful partnerships is mindfulness. Just as precious gems acquired one-by-one can be assembled into a necklace, Section 4 shows you how to create a support circle one relationship at a time with conscious intent. In this section, you'll learn how shifting your perspective rights your relationships. The small steps include a reflection on your readiness to ask for help along with the skills and strategies for *consciously cultivating* a circle of peer mentors, peer editors, co-presenters, co-authors, and partners.

Your Nurse–Companions

Because disillusionment with past collaborations can leave nurses reluctant to ask for peer mentoring or editing, it may not surprise you to read that a few of your nurse–companions have reservations about cultivating a support circle. When asked how the idea of cultivating support circles of colleague–friends sounds, this is what each wrote:

Keri's free-write reads:

> To be honest, and it's kind of embarrassing to admit, I'm leery about partnerships with nursing colleagues. While I grew up in a communal culture, as a nurse practitioner I've had to learn to function as an independent agent. Even hearing that word—partnerships—dredges up memories of group projects where, to keep my 'A' average, I carried the deadweight of fellow students only too happy to let me do their part of our project for them. So I'm going to have to work hard at keeping a beginner's mind as I read this section.

Betty wrote:

> In my personal life, I've got lots of support circles, like my quilting group and my garden club. Reading Sections II and III made me realize how much of a giver I am in my professional life. Even though sometimes I wish someone would peer mentor or edit my work the way I do theirs, asking for help isn't easy for me. When it comes right down to it, I'm pretty much of a perfectionist. I worry I'd exhaust anyone who tried to peer mentor me, which is why I liked that three-question approach to peer editing. My peer editor asked me three questions, and I went to town with revising my newsletter manuscript without bothering him again.

Justin writes:

> I'm pretty good at creating support circles. When you grow up in a big family like I did, I guess it comes naturally. I've got colleague–friends who will be happy to peer mentor and peer edit my stuff, which is a good thing, because I'm drafting a manuscript from my poster presentation for the *Men in Nursing Magazine.* Now that I want to get involved at the national level in the "American Association for Men in Nursing," I'm looking to add a mentor to my support circle. Someone with the political savvy and connections to help me assume leadership positions that will make a difference for men in nursing education.

It's understandable that classmates who didn't carry their weight left Keri reticent about creating a support circle. Meanwhile, Betty and Justin are considering the type of assistance they'd like from colleague–friends and mentors. Now that you've read their free-writes, it's time for you to answer the same question (see Jot Box 80-1).

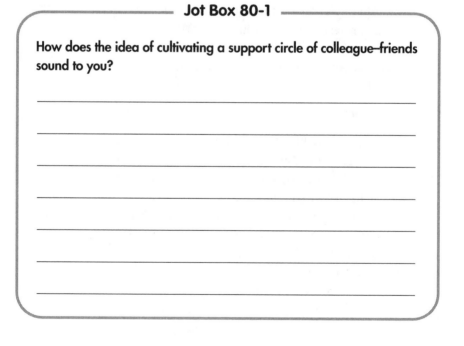

Jot Box 80-1

How does the idea of cultivating a support circle of colleague–friends sound to you?

Whether you'd like to create a support circle from scratch or you've got one that you'd like to compare with mine, read on.

TIP

Colleague–friends can infuse your professional life with an exuberant mix of camaraderie and competence.

Reference

1. Heinrich, K. T., Pardue, K., Davison-Price, M., Murphy, J. I., Neese, R., Walker, P., & White, K. B. (2005). How can I help you? How can you help me? Transforming nursing education through partnerships. *Nursing Education Perspectives, 26*(1), 34–41.

I Reach Out and Receive with Gratitude

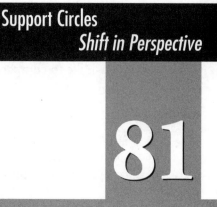

Piglet sidled up to Pooh from behind.
"Pooh," he whispered.
"Yes, Piglet?"
"Nothing," said Piglet, taking Pooh's paw,
"I just wanted to be sure of you."

A. A. Milne

Reading *Winnie the Pooh* not long ago reminded me that a child's life is full of asking for help. When caught in a predicament, A. A. Milne's ensemble cast of animal characters—Pooh, Piglet, Eeyore, Rabbit—and their boy-pal Christopher Robin carefully consider who to ask for help. Why, if asking for help is child's play, is it so hard for nurses to do? Judging from our reluctance to ask for help, you'd think that a renegade fairy allowed nurses three wishes per lifetime. Not wanting to waste a one, we stifle our yearnings and keep our mouths shut.

In dark moments, when you're too tuckered out to care anymore, do you ever ask yourself why it's you who's always doing the giving? The only way to change this is to *shift your perspective* from going it alone to reaching out for help. How? By practicing three fine arts: knowing what you need, asking for help, and receiving with grace. To see just how much practice it's going to take, this chapter poses three questions.

First, how are you at taking care of your needs? To see, over the next day or so respond to your needs as they arise. When you become aware that you're hungry, eat. Need a bathroom break, take it now. If you rarely respond to your physical needs, you're used to overriding messages from your body. Becoming aware of your needs as they arise is good practice for knowing what you'll be needing for your dare-to-share projects. Then it will be easier to answer the two questions posed in Jot Box 81-1.

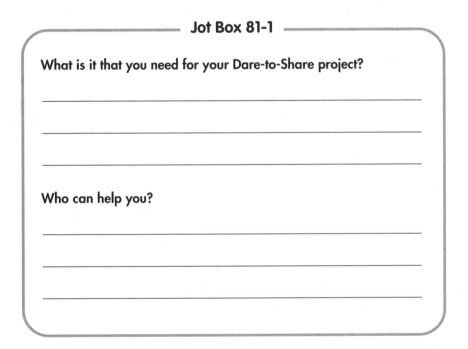

Jot Box 81-1

What is it that you need for your Dare-to-Share project?

_____

_____

_____

Who can help you?

_____

_____

_____

Be patient with yourself. When you're used to repressing your professional needs and desires, it may take some time to figure out what it is you need. With practice, getting in touch with your needs will take less and less time. Knowing what you need makes it easier to ask for help.

Speaking of, how are you at asking for help? To become part of a support circle, you must learn to reach out—even when, like Piglet, all you need is a touch of reassurance because you're feeling a bit insecure. To see where you are on the "Asking for Help Continuum," think about the last time you wanted or needed help in your professional life, especially if it related to a dare-to-share challenge. Keep this event in mind as you mark your place on the continuum below.

Always Ask	Sometimes Ask	Never Ask
1	5	10

The "Ask For Help" Continuum

If your score is closer to 10 than to 1, you've got some practicing to do.

Sometimes receiving can even be harder than asking for help. How are you with accepting compliments? If you shrug them off or act as if you don't hear them, anything to brush them off so your head doesn't get too big, consider this. Taking compliments is the same skill as opening yourself up to all the good things in life. So the next time someone gives you a compliment, practice the gentle art of gratitude. Allow those kind words to sink in, like daffodils raising their sweet yellow faces to drops of rain from a spring shower. Receiving is as much a part of peer mentoring and peer editing as asking for help.

During this section, try something different. Commit to reaching out and receiving as open-handedly as you give. Then, as you dare to share, you'll find yourself overflowing with gratitude for the colleague–friends who give as much as they get from you.

TIP

Don't go it alone! Know what you need, ask for help and receive with gratitude.

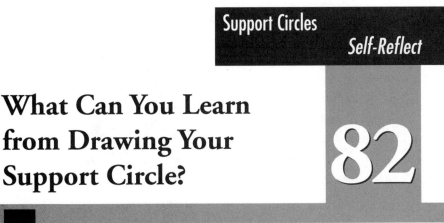

What Can You Learn from Drawing Your Support Circle?

82

> *The form of the circle itself is an embodiment of wisdom . . . when a circle is taken into the workplace or community . . . it enhances collaborative undertakings and brings people who work together emotionally closer and in a less hierarchical relationship to one another.*

Jean Shinoda Bolen

When Molly and Christina, my peer editors, suggested that we draw our support circles in this chapter, I was intrigued enough to go home and draw mine. After identifying a specific work-smart project, this is how my circle looked for my *Dare to Share* writing project (see Figure 82-1).

What an exercise in gratitude! As I wrote the name of each supporter into the circle, I thanked him or her for a special contribution to this project. Writing "Me" into the center of support circles serves as a reminder to recognize your own contributions, because, regardless of the project, you are your biggest supporter. My list grew over the course

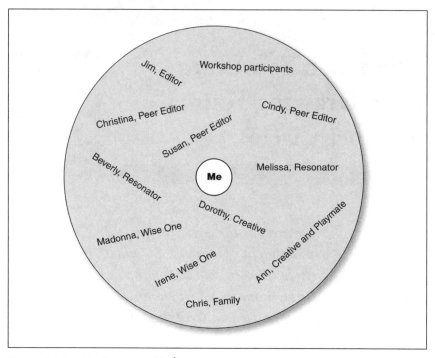

Figure 82-1   My Support Circle
My Dare to Share Project: When the Joy Stealer is Me

of a few days as I kept remembering the names of people to add. Drawing my support circle gave me three new insights:

1. My circle grew one relationship at a time.
2. I didn't set out to assemble a support circle, it just happened.
3. They all know me without necessarily knowing each other.

After I'd completed my list, I grouped my various supporters by the roles they played and assigned each grouping a descriptive title. "Colleague–Friends & Resonators" included the workshop participants along with the editor, peer editors, and colleagues who'd helped me to refine my ideas—Jim, Christina, Susan, Cindy, Melissa, and Beverly; "Creatives & Playmates" included the women who'd given me insights through movement or during artistic activities—Dorothy and Ann; "Wise Ones & Mentors" included two wise women who own their "inner joy-stealer" with grace—Irene and Madonna; and, "Family & Friends" included my

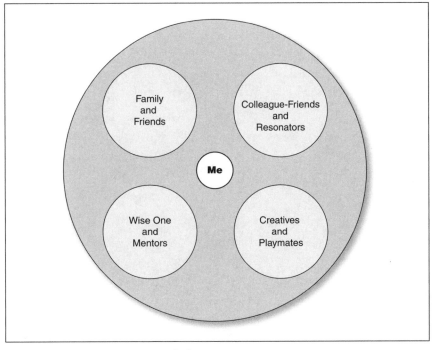

Figure 82-2   My Support Circle by Grouping

significant other who owns his inner joy-stealer and helps me to own mine—Chris.

Looking at my four groupings—colleague–friends and resonators, creatives and playmates, wise ones and mentors, and family and friends—I began to see how each person entered my life when needed most. Although no one person is the whole package, together they form a kaleidoscope that colors my project with just the right splashes of exuberance, compassion, and reality checks. We dance in and out of one another's lives, sometimes in one role, at other times in another, depending on what's happening. In between, we never lose our fondness for one another or our willingness to drop what we're doing to help each other.

It's time for you to draw your support circle of colleague–friends for a dare-to-share project (see Figure 82-3). So you don't forget to add the biggest supporter of your project, there's a "Me" already written into the center of the circle.

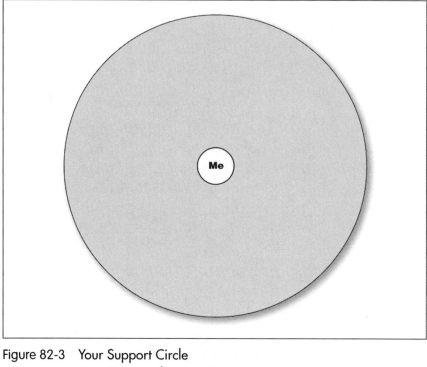

Figure 82-3 Your Support Circle
Your Dare to Share Project: _____

How was that for you? If you haven't given much thought to this, you may find yourself adding the names of other supporters to your drawing over the next few days and weeks. Once you feel like you've pretty much included everyone, group them according to the roles they play in your support circle and assign a descriptive name to each grouping (see Figure 82-4).

Don't be upset if your support circle looks a bit skimpy. If cultivating a support circle is a new concept, give yourself some time to develop a cadre of colleague–friends. Katharine White, my colleague–friend and life coach, was the first person who taught me about "support teams." Whenever I'd tell her about a challenge I was facing, the first question she'd ask is who can help you with this. Nine out of 10 times, I drew a blank. But as I thought more about it, someone would come to mind or appear within a few days or weeks. While my original circle grew itself over the years, by asking myself Katharine's question with each new

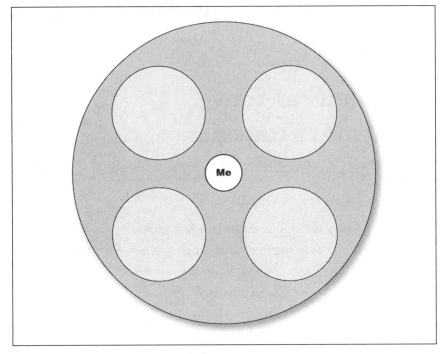

Figure 82-4   Your Support Circle by Grouping

project, I now add to my support circle with mindfulness. For those of you who would like to develop or expand your support circle with mindfulness, the next chapters offer lots of clues and tips.

TIP

Be grateful to those in your support circle who help you manifest your dare-to-share projects.

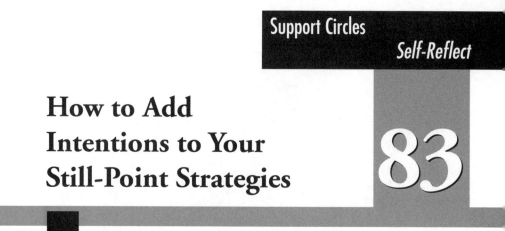

How to Add Intentions to Your Still-Point Strategies

83

Only when one is connected to one's inner core is one connected to others. And, for me, the core, the inner spring, can best be re-found through solitude.

Anne Morrow Lindbergh

When driving home from the airport following a consultation visit at 2:00 A.M., a policeman pulled me over. No wonder it seemed darker than usual; I was driving without headlights. After a half hour spent contacting AAA for a tow and calling home for a ride, the policeman asked me to give my headlights one last try. This time they went on full power. I canceled AAA and called Chris to tell him to go back to sleep. Back on the road again, I couldn't believe what a difference those head-lights made. Without them, it was easy to get confused on a familiar road. With them, it was like driving home in the light of day.

Adding an intention to your still-point strategy is like turning on your headlights. Like all actions, still-point strategies flow from inten-tions. *Intentions* are wishes or requests. Author and medical-intuitive Carolyn Myss suggests using the phrase "I am open to . . ." to introduce intentions.[1] One of her intentions for creativity reads, "I am open to receiving guidance on how to proceed with my work" (p. 303).[1]

Whether praying for divine intervention or considering who in your circles can help with your next dare-to-share step, adding conscious intentions to still-point strategies makes them even more purposeful.

Let me give you an example. One of my favorite still-point strategies is lighting a candle. Before I light the candle, I take my creative task into consideration. If this is a day when I need to brainstorm ideas for a presentation, I set an intention—"I am open to inspiration"—and light my candle. As you can see in the following box, my task for today is revising this section, so using the same still-point strategy, I set a different intention.

My Task, Intention, and Still-Point Strategy

My creative task: Revise Section 4 of *Dare to Share*.

My intention: I am open to the beginner's mind necessary for revising this section with clarity and patience.

My still-point strategy: Light a candle.

Even though I dragged myself out of bed and into my study this morning because I wasn't in the mood for revising, expressing my request for beginner's mind is helping me to focus on my creative task with clarity and patience.

Now it's your turn. Consider your creative task for today. Say it's reading the next chapter in this section. What intention will help you complete your task? You may want to use one of the four *shifts in perspective* from earlier sections to craft your intention to open to creativity—beginner's mind, working smart, or reaching out and receiving help. Insert your responses into Jot Box 83-1.

Practice the following three steps: contemplate your task, set your intention, and enact a still-point strategy. Once your task is completed, see what a difference adding an intention to your still point made. If this combo allows you to make better use of your creative time, you might want to make these three steps a habit. Now, if you're open to adding peer mentors to your support circle, you'll want to read Beverly Sastri's description of our peer-mentoring experiences in the next storytelling chapter.

Jot Box 83-1

Your Task, Intention, and Still-Point Strategy

Your creative task:

_____

Your intention: I am open to

_____

Your still-point strategy:

_____

TIP

Light the way for your creative tasks by adding intentions to your still-point strategies.

References

1. Myss, C. (2001). *Sacred contracts: Awakening your divine potential.* New York: Harmony Books.

How to Put the Pizzazz in Peer-Mentoring Partnerships

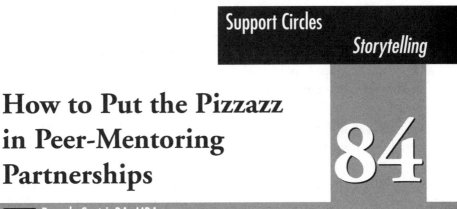

84

Beverly Sastri, BA, MBA

> *"To be" is first of all to be visible. So we*
> *seek lovers and mentors and friends that*
> *we may be seen, and blessed.*

James Hillman

Imagine having a magic genie in your life: someone who has all the answers; makes sure your life stays on track; and, as needed, works a charm that makes you more vibrant, confident, productive, and joyful. Imagine someone who helps you resolve the frustrations, doubts, and fears that hold you back in the process of reviewing and improving our dare-to-share projects. And finally, imagine being so in tune that this person can even listen for what you *don't* say and respond to that! Your genie awaits: She or he is called a peer mentor.

Looking for a New Tennis Partner

My initiation into peer mentoring began with a chance meeting. I belonged to a support circle that consisted of women who were all at the same level of development and experience. Knowing that improving your tennis game means playing with those at a higher skill level, I started looking for a new "tennis partner" who would challenge me to grow.

After seeing Kathy present at the Association of Women Business Leaders (AWBL) meeting, I spoke with her because I was struck by her obvious mastery of her topic material as well as by her down-to-earth, engaging presentation style. We agreed to meet for lunch, but months passed, and we never got around to it. The next time I saw Kathy at an AWBL meeting, I marched over and said, "Get out your calendar—this time we really *are* going to have lunch!"

Our initial getting-to-know-you meeting went very well, and we agreed to try on a peer-mentoring partnership. It was clear that I could benefit from Kathy's experience with presenting and publishing and she could profit from my "Create a Life You Love" training as well as my business and marketing background. Based on my previous experience of peer mentoring, I assumed this meant we would meet occasionally, bring each other up-to-date on our current projects, focus on a given area or problem, and then make "promises" as to what we would do before our next meeting. Little did I know! Kathy proceeded to introduce me to a turbo-charged version of peer mentoring that included contracting upfront by specifying what type of support we were seeking, how often we would meet, and what format our meetings would follow.

Contracting and Re-Contracting

At first we agreed to meet once a week for an hour and to alternate the focus: the hour would be Kathy's one week and mine the next. It quickly became apparent that this wasn't enough frequency, and we decided to meet twice each week, one hour per person. It's amazing to think that we've been meeting this way for four years. Over that time, we've refined our interaction style and problem-solving skills to the point where we cover twice as much material with the same level of ease. Our meeting format ensures that each of us stays in role. When it's not "your" meeting, be an active listener, let the other person lead the conversation, and keep your input clear and concise.

An added plus is the spontaneous ways a peer-mentoring relationship can evolve. We've added semi-annual meetings, one in January to establish our vision and goals and one in June to revisit and set new visions or goals if necessary. To accommodate needs that arise between our weekly meetings, as a safety net when something unexpected and time-driven pops up, we e-mail requests with a specific description of the type of assistance needed as well as a due date. The sender follows up with a phone message calling attention to the request. Importantly, it is understood that each of us has an automatic "get out of jail free" card—the option to refuse any request if it's too difficult to respond within the allotted time. Neither of us has ever abused this privilege, which speaks to the level of sensitivity and mutual respect inherent in our peer-mentoring relationship.

Our most recent renegotiation occurred when we realized our sessions had become so focused on our projects that we had no time to acknowledge the internal transformations happening along the way. So we set aside an extra meeting devoted entirely to sharing our own and appreciating each other's personal growth stories. Let me tell you, reflective time-outs like this don't happen often enough in our lives.

Giving You a Peek into Our Sessions

To give you a sense of what it's like to "do" peer mentoring, here are a few snapshots from our sessions. As a Sage presenter, I wasn't comfortable asking questions of the audience because I didn't know what they'd say. It took a great deal of coaching from my Guide mentor, in addition to watching her engage audience participants, before I began to experiment with putting the "show" ahead of the "tell." The difference is as astonishing as it is simple. These days, rather than launching into a lecture, my presentations open with an exercise or a story. Now that I know that it's the audience's willingness to share that truly brings a presentation to life, I ask, "What was that like for you?" Their answers make my topic fresh and relevant in a way I never could on my own. By turning audiences into participants, I am gifted with new insights that allow me to expand my material. When I realized that I *prefer* engaging the audience, I knew my Sage style had stretched to include Guide-like qualities.

Beyond changing how I present, peer mentoring has given me a systematic approach to the entire process of presenting. Kathy's Presentation Worksheet forces me to be clear about who is my audience, what is my purpose, and what response I'm seeking. It's amazing how many times I think I know these answers in advance only to discover an eye-glittering idea or snappy slant because I forced myself to take the time to fill out the Presentation Worksheet. This worksheet becomes my touchstone and compass as I develop the presentation. It's easier than you might think to wander off slant in the excitement of the moment. Reviewing presentations with Kathy in peer mentoring pre-sessions allows us to smooth the rough spots, check overall flow and timing, and make sure it passes the slant test.

After each presentation, no matter how large or small, I collate audience evaluations comments and complete my What Worked & Future Changes Worksheet. I'm always astounded at how little time it takes to do this and how many ah-hahs come to light that I might otherwise miss. Sharing these, along with getting Kathy's observations during my post-session, invariably deepens my insights. Afterwards I summarize all the refinements and file them with that workshop's materials. Before developing the next worksheet and presentation, I review recent post-session evaluation materials to make sure I apply the lessons learned.

Peer mentoring helps as much with calming the voice of my inner critic as with developing and evaluating presentations. Last fall I committed to doing a series of radio interviews based on the human-potential work I teach. As soon as I made the commitment and began booking interviews, panic struck. Convinced I was going to sound like an idiot on air, I brought my fears to my next peer-mentoring session. Our conversation made me realize that I was focused on the wrong thing. I was more concerned about sounding good than I was on communicating the concepts clearly and accurately. That realization not only dispelled my concerns, but also restored the energy and passion I feel for this work.

Enriching Our Partnership with Our Differences

Because partnerships are reciprocal, well-chosen peer mentors benefit each other by sharing their unique backgrounds, experiences, skills, and perspectives. It is our differences, even more than our similarities, that enrich our partnership. Kathy's training as a psychotherapist, educator, and author has given me new tools for dealing with tough clients and creating standout presentations. My background as a business owner, corporate marketer, and consultant on human potential have helped Kathy improve her entrepreneurial skills and envision and create a work life she loves.

Our psychological and style differences also are a perfect complement. I am comfortable with and even energized by deadlines, timelines, and a fairly rigid structure to my day. Kathy works equally hard, but in a less structured way. She has taught me how to go with the flow more and balance my productive outbursts with creative, restful, and/or physical activities that recharge my batteries, reduce stress, and actually increase my productivity. As a Sage presenter, I have taught Kathy how to become more comfortable in the spotlight. As a Guide on the Side she has taught me the joy of letting the collective wisdom of the audience guide the direction of a workshop or presentation.

In looking back over our peer-mentoring relationship, I am awed by how much our partnership contributes to my business and personal growth. In addition to sharing our skills and experiences, we keep each other on track. At the beginning of each peer-mentoring session, we speak our goals and visions aloud. It's very difficult to "hide out" when you're meeting with someone every week and they are completely up to speed on what you have committed to create. Our respect, impeccability, and openness has addicted me to this level of high-quality relationship. Over time, I have not only created other peer-mentoring relationships, I am transforming my personal friendships into this same level of support and interaction. Life becomes very rich when everyone in your social circle is also a member of your support circle. They know what your current personal and work goals are and stand ready to support you with whatever feedback, ideas, or resources you may need.

Conclusion

Once experienced, peer-mentoring partnerships may become one of life's gifts that you're no longer willing to live without. I recently met a woman at a party. After discovering we were both "solopreneurs" with complementary interests, we decided to meet and begin sharing our experiences and expertise. Now it was her turn to become nonplussed when, without even thinking, I began talking about contracting and establishing our peer-mentoring protocol. Like me, she had previously only experienced a less formal version. At her request, we kept things more informal at first, but once she began to experience the added value peer mentoring brings to her business and her overall state of mind, she asked to establish a more structured schedule and format for meetings.

I'll always have peer mentors in my support circle because:

1. They stimulate an inspired level of thought and creativity.
2. They enrich my life with their diversity of experience, perspective, and skills.
3. They believe in my greatness and won't let me sell myself short.
4. They acknowledge and celebrate my strengths and successes.
5. They support me in viewing my weaknesses and failures so that I learn from both.
6. They hold me to my word to keep me on task and on track.
7. They provide a safe space to identify and release self-judgments and fears.
8. They help me understand where I am stuck and why.
9. They remind me of the big picture when I am mired in detail.
10. They share my excitement over what I am creating in my life.

These are 10 good reasons to consider peer mentoring when facing your next dare-to-share challenge.

TIP
Power up your next presentation with the help of a peer mentor.

How to Check if Creative Collaborations Pass the Zest Test

85

> *We do not believe in ourselves until someone reveals that deep inside of us something is valuable, worth listening to, worthy of our trust, sacred to our touch. Once we believe in ourselves we can risk curiosity, wonder, spontaneous delight, or any experience that reveals the human spirit.*
>
> e.e. cummings

How is it that after four years of meeting twice a week Beverly and I still leave our sessions feeling exuberant? Jean Baker Miller would say that ours, like all "mutually created and mutually enhancing, empathetic relationships . . . generate a greater sense of energy or zest, knowledge of self and other, capacity to act, sense of self-worth and desire for further connection" (p. 12).[1] Jean Shinoda Bolen might explain it as a chemical response. Scientists are discovering that the rush women get from relating to one another in meaningful ways comes from the release of the hormone oxytocin.[2] Philosopher Martin Buber[3] might attribute our exuberance to an "I–thou" relationship in which people feel seen for who they are, while neuroscientists like Louis Cozolino[4] would say that brains are hardwired for relational connections such as ours.

369

Whatever the explanation, eye glitter is contagious when partnerships are zestful. To see if your relationship with a colleague–friend passes the "Zest Test," check off the items that apply to the relationship in Jot Box 85-1.

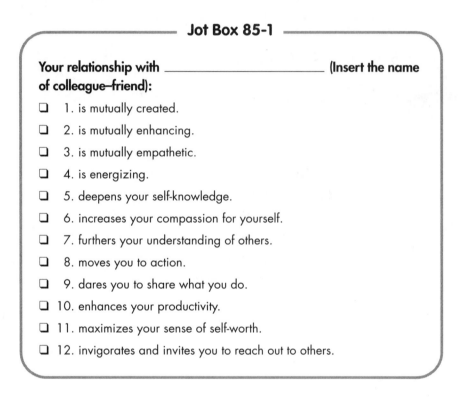

Jot Box 85-1

Your relationship with _____ **(Insert the name of colleague–friend):**

❏ 1. is mutually created.

❏ 2. is mutually enhancing.

❏ 3. is mutually empathetic.

❏ 4. is energizing.

❏ 5. deepens your self-knowledge.

❏ 6. increases your compassion for yourself.

❏ 7. furthers your understanding of others.

❏ 8. moves you to action.

❏ 9. dares you to share what you do.

❏ 10. enhances your productivity.

❏ 11. maximizes your sense of self-worth.

❏ 12. invigorates and invites you to reach out to others.

If you checked 10 out of 12 of the items, your relationship passes the Zest Test with flying colors. Don't settle for less in your creative collaborations! If you're finding your relationship with collaborators on a presentation or publication project less than zestful, your collaborators are probably feeling the same way. In the next storytelling chapter, two colleague–friends, Christina Purpora and Molly Davison-Price, reveal what they've learned about making peer-editing relationships a zestful collaboration.

■ **TIP**
Choose your colleague–friends for the zest they add to your life.

References

1. Baker Miller, J. (1986). What do we mean by relationships? *Work-in-Progress, No. 22*. Wellesley, MA: Stone Center Working Paper Series.
2. Shinoda Bolen, J. (2005). *Urgent message from MOTHER: Gather the women, save the world*. York, ME: Conari Press.
3. Buber, M. (2006). *I and thou*. London: Hespirides Press.
4. Cozolino, L. (2006). *The neuroscience of human relationships*. New York: W. W. Norton.

How to Trade an Editor's Red Pen for a Peer Editor's Compassion

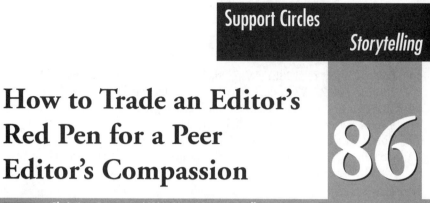

86

Christina Purpora, MSN, RN, CCRN & Molly Davison-Price, RN, MSN

May the sun bring you new energy by day.
May the moon softly restore you by night,
May the rain wash away your worries,
May the breeze blow new strength into your being.
May you walk gently through the world and
know its beauty all the days of your life.

Apache blessing

When Kathy asked us to peer edit a book she was writing on presenting and publishing, we felt prepared to accept because we'd been peer editors in the past. Not only that! We knew that our backgrounds as clinicians and educators qualified us as members of the *Dare to Share* readership *and* ensured that our feedback would keep this book true to nurse-readers. As hoped, our peer-editing partnership proved to be a mutually supportive and intellectually stimulating adventure. We felt much less prepared when Kathy dared us to share by writing a chapter about our peer-editing experience. Because we'd never before collaborated on a writing project, we did what we'd learned to do as peer editors. We asked questions. Only this time we answered them, too. To share what we've learned about good peer editing, this chapter poses the six questions that we asked each other, shares our answers, and follows each question and answer with an insight.

Reflections on Being Edited

Once we realized how much our past experiences with editing influenced our responses to peer editing, we asked ourselves what was it like to have our own writing edited.

Molly: My experiences with teachers who reviewed my drafts with red pens go way back. Even my mother would cross out my ideas as she would "help" me with my papers in high school. It felt like an annihilation of my ideas. Because this was my experience of having a paper edited, when I reviewed someone else's paper and the ideas did not flow, my red pen took over. Crossing out the writer's ideas, I'd rewrite the paper. When I finally looked up, I'd see the same dejected look on the writer's face that I used to get when my mother crossed out my words with her red pen. Then I'd feel terrible for being insensitive.

Christina: When I started peer editing Kathy's manuscript, I was still fixing words on the page. I had an intellectual understanding of peer editing; I wasn't yet able to put it into practice. Even while clinging to that familiar red pen, I felt uncomfortable. The "red-pen maniac editors" in my life were the nuns from my Catholic boarding school days and a few undergraduate teachers. Red pens in hand, they would slash sentences, cutting the glimmers from my inspirations. When I got back what I'd written, I'd get a lump in my throat as I turned to the first page of the paper. Feeling that familiar sense of disappointment and unable to see beyond the red, I wanted the readers of my work to lose their pens. I wanted them to share their feelings and thoughts with me about what I'd written.

Our unhappy memories turned into catalysts as experiences like these led to our wanting to change our approaches to editing.

Insight #1: Being a good peer editor means remembering what it feels like to have a red-pen maniac edit your writing.

Reflections on Lessons Learned from Experienced Peer Editors

We agreed that we'd learned more from observing peer editing than from all of the how-to instructions in our graduate program. So we asked each other, "What have you learned from watching more experienced peer editors?"

Molly: When I was a part of an eight-person team that co-presented and co-published an article, we were individually e-mailed each draft of the manuscript to peer edit. We e-mailed our thoughts to one another about how to make it better. One idea in the draft seemed foggy to me; others in the group concurred. Being the least-experienced peer editor, I watched as they handled their confusion by saying, "This idea is interesting, I'd like to know more about this." Comments like this opened the dialogue around the confusion while maintaining the connectedness in our relationship. I was so relieved I hadn't hit the send button with my "this doesn't make any sense" comment, which would have closed the dialogue and possibly hurt the relationship. When we were together, there was a feeling of great support and respect for each member of the team that was infectious. I liked how it felt to be a member of this support circle. Seeing others giving feedback to each other in an honest and supportive way improved my skills as a peer editor.

Christina: My first group experience with peer editing was when Molly and I peer edited *Dare to Share* for Kathy. At our meetings, I noticed that we didn't get right to business. Instead we took time to connect with each other, sharing what was going on in our personal and professional lives. When we actually started the process of peer editing, I noticed Kathy and Molly engaged in a dialogue. Molly asked questions to clarify her confusion and Kathy, in turn, asked questions to clarify her understanding of Molly's feedback. Instead of Molly's handing over pages bleeding with red pen marks, it was Kathy who wrote notes on her pad of paper.

Insight #2: Being a good peer editor means learning the art of asking questions from more experienced peer editors.

Reflections on Respecting the Author–Peer Editor Relationship

Committed to mending our ways, we reflected on what's missing from the red-pen approach by asking each other, "How does your feedback respect the author–peer editor relationship?"

Molly: Seeing the author as a person reframes the job of peer editing. Now I begin each session with questions for the author: Why *do you* want to write this? What message are you trying to convey? Who is the audience you're trying to reach? Then I listen patiently to the responses and ask for more clarification when ideas remain unclear. Careful listening increases my ability to ask questions that provide clarity. I find that asking questions and listening to the answers to form new questions develops trusting relationships with authors.

Christina: When I give feedback, connecting with the author is in the forefront of my mind as well. I begin by saying something positive—an overall statement of what I felt as I read the piece. I believe it's important to say that I love the work if I do. By listening, paying attention to visual and verbal cues, I pick up signals from the author's body language and words about what feedback is helpful and what is not so helpful. With that understood, I'll provide specifics about what I'm wanting as a reader, for example, more information or less? This give-and-take honors our relationship.

Insight #3: Being a good peer editor means giving feedback in ways that foster trusting relationships with authors.

Reflections on What's Needed to Peer Edit

Peer editing is a big responsibility that we both took seriously. Although we were both reviewing the same document, we each had our own way of going about peer editing. So we asked each other, "What did you need to get the job done?"

Molly: When going about the actual work of peer editing, I've heeded Kathy's advice to use a still-point strategy which, in my case, is a cup of tea to get me into a creative mood. I know I'll need to read the manuscript several times. Hence, I set aside a big block of time without other deadlines and commitments hanging over me. Taking notes about the questions I want to ask helps me stay focused while reading the manuscript and gives me a list to refer to during our face-to-face meeting.

Christina: To give my undivided attention to reading, I need to feel quiet. So my still-point strategy is to turn off all sources of sound, such as phones, to avoid potential interruptions. After doing this, I feel relaxed and ready to focus when I sit down in the corner of my couch to read. I also need enough time to read the piece through three times. Because this is a serious time commitment, I make an appointment with myself to read the manuscript. This allows me to stay focused and balance my commitment to Kathy with other responsibilities in my life.

Insight #4: Being a good peer editor means knowing what to do to create the proper conditions to complete the task.

Reflections on the Surprises

It's sometimes hard to know what you're getting yourself into when you say yes to a peer editing relationship. When we asked each other, was there anything that you didn't expect in your peer editing relationship, our answer was the same.

Molly and Christina: Peer-editing relationships require flexibility as the project unfolds. Although we originally agreed to a time frame of three to four months, we soon realized that this project was going to require more time, so we renegotiated our conditions (e.g., the schedule of meeting times and the volume of material we could read at any one time). When we started the project, our contract was completing our "job" as peer editors. As time progressed, our relationship deepened from that of a job to an investment in Kathy's completing *Dare to Share* for you.

Insight #5: Being a good peer editor means staying flexible and renegotiating PRN.

Reflections on the Benefits for the Peer Editor

As we discovered, peer editing is not just a favor you do for a colleague–friend. To learn more about the hidden treasures for peer editors, we asked each other, "What did you get from peer editing?"

Molly: Kathy's finding my input thought provoking was thrill enough; who knew that peer editing would turn on my creative juices. The opportunity to watch an accomplished writer prepare a book manuscript was invaluable to me as a hopeful writer. I've always loved talking about two of my passions, nursing and education; our discussions reminded me that my ideas are valuable enough to write about. During our connecting time at the beginning of each peer-editing session, Kathy and Christina offered advice that helped me make decisions about my teaching career with a "yes, you can and go for it" attitude. This allowed Christina and me to reestablish a dialogue about interests we hope to pursue together.

Christina: My understanding of peer editing has grown through this experience. Our peer-editing circle was a safe place for me to test out new ways of editing. I've learned, for example, to read a manuscript from the point of view of the readers. Sometimes, for example, when Kathy used certain phrases or words, my gut would tighten. I'd explore my feeling as a reader a bit more so that when I gave Kathy feedback about how I felt, I could put my gut reaction into words. During our peer-editing session, I'd ask Kathy for clarification about what she'd written so that I could understand what she meant. Becoming aware of my thoughts and feelings allowed me to offer authentic feedback from a reader's point of view in a sensitive manner. By being in a support circle with Kathy and Molly, I am transforming the red-pen-maniac editor within into a receptive and responsive peer editor who dialogues with colleague–friends.

Insight #6: Being a good peer editor means getting as well as giving!

Conclusion

It's all too easy to edit as you've been edited. The more we learn about what it means to be a good peer editor, the better we are at disarming the red-pen maniac within. No more crushers of creativity, as recovering red-pen maniacs who continue to grow and evolve into insightful peer editors, we are members of a support circle that sparks inspiration and innovation. Feel free to use our questions, answers, and insights as a starting point if you want to trade your red pen for the compassionate insights of a peer editor. We're rooting for you!

TIP
Drop the red pen and enjoy the creative collaboration that is peer editing.

What's a Resonator?

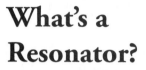

If you obey all the rules, you miss all the fun.

Katharine Hepburn

I got much, much more than I asked for by breaking the rule of one peer editor per writing project. As a two-some, I knew that Molly and Christina were the perfect peer editors for *Dare to Share*. What I didn't know was that we would over this last year become resonators for each other. A resonator is:

> A friend or a sister or companion so true to her own inner reality that she inspires [us] to be faithful to [ours]. Somehow the resonator calls us to our true selves, reminding us and reflecting to us our deepest possibility, asking the difficult questions and encouraging us to take action (p. 209).[1]

After I share how we fulfilled these resonator roles in our peer-editing partnership, you'll get the chance to do the same with your colleague–friends.

Reminding and reflecting to us our deepest possibility. Never mind butterflies, I felt like Lear jets were zooming around in my stomach as I drove to our first meeting. Molly and Christina were the first people who'd ever read my chapter drafts. Terrified about what they'd say, my inner critic had been dancing a jig atop my self-esteem. My darkest fear was that I didn't have what it takes to write a book, so when Christina's first words were, "I loved it," relief washed over me.

Asking the difficult questions. With unerring accuracy, Molly's questions have always punctured my assumptions and backlit the holes in my thinking. That's why I asked her to peer edit *Dare to Share*. From our first meeting, a pattern was set. Christina's expression of appreciation relaxed me so that by the time Molly got around to asking questions such as who *is* my audience and what *is* my voice, I might not be able to answer, but at least I could hear the questions. After mulling over her latest question, I'd finally get what Molly was asking with barely enough time to revise my draft for our next session. Then she'd ask her next question and another six weeks would go by before I had an answer. Without Molly's perceptive questions and Christina's creative suggestions, *Dare to Share* wouldn't be the answer to your questions.

Encouraging us to take action. Each of us has grown from our dialogues about our dreams and our fears. In a year's time, Christina has become one of the five fellows accepted to the University of California at San Francisco's doctoral program; Molly has taught two courses as an adjunct faculty person and is exploring options for her next teaching challenge; and I'm finishing a book I wasn't even sure I could write.

When I said I got much more than I asked for, I meant it. Over the last year, we've met every four to six weeks for editorial review sessions. By my deadline, Molly and Christina will each have clocked 150 hours in editing and feedback sessions. We had already far exceeded my initial estimate of the time and the number of meetings involved by the time they offered to read the entire manuscript before it was submitted to the publisher.

So now that you know what a resonator is, who in your professional life asks you questions that leave you playing with answers for days afterwards? Who allows you to come upon the answers in your own time? Who listens in a way that you feel heard as well as seen? (See Jot Box 87-1.)

Consider yourself blessed if you have a colleague–friend(s) who are resonators in your support circle. If you don't yet have a resonator in your professional life, put the word out. You may, in time, recognize a colleague–friend who's been there all along or someone new will come into your life. In the next chapter, you'll read about the Cosmic Connection, three colleague–friends, whose resonating partnership calls them to scale new heights both individually and as a group on a regular basis.

=================== **Jot Box 87-1** ===================

Resonator Questionnaire

Who do you have in your life who:

Reminds you and reflects your deepest possibility to you?

_____

Ask the difficult questions?

_____

Encourages you to take action?

_____

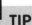

TIP

Treasure the resonators in your life whether they're walk-on's or stick-arounds.

Reference

1. Anderson, S. R., & Hopkins, P. (1991). *The feminine face of god.* New York: Bantam.

What Are Three Words That Turn Competitions into Collaborations?

88

Kathleen T. Heinrich, RN, PhD, Cynthia Clark, RN, PhD, and Susan Luparell, RN, PhD

*There are no shortcuts to
any place worth going.*

Anonymous

As in sports, so in nursing. Competition can enliven and strengthen. Or it can splinter colleague–friendships, steal joy, and leave those involved fallen by the wayside or limping to a finish line where there are no winners. Three competitive and hard-working nurse presenters and authors, Kathy, Cindy, and Susan (we), process issues and collaborate on groundbreaking projects that in many other groups might cause rivalry and conflict. After trekking into the unexplored, relational terrain of partnerships, we discovered that the secret for keeping our connection cosmic is three little words—*yours, mine,* and *ours.* If you yearn to share what you do in ways that invigorate rather than alienate your collaborators, this chapter shows how these words can galvanize your relationships with colleague–friends.

Our Story

Cindy and Susan are nurse educators who live in the Western mountain states. Cindy is a professor at Boise State University, and Susan is an assistant professor at Montana State University. Along with Kathy, we call

381

ourselves the "Cosmic Connection," and our partnership began two years ago. Our shared interest in researching incivility to cultivate civility in nursing education brought us together. What keeps us together is our commitment to working through feelings of envy, anger, and competition[1] in ways that allow us to celebrate our own and each other's success.

Although incivility is defined as "showing disregard and insolence for others causing an atmosphere of disrespect, conflict, and stress;"[2] civility is "Respect for others, a willingness to hear each other's views, and the exercise of restraint in criticizing the views and actions of others."[3] Because our experiences are initiating us into new ways of relating, this chapter uses the three stages in the hero's journey—the call to adventure, the initiation and the return—to structure our story.

The heroic quest, according to Joseph Campbell,[4] is a metaphor for an uncertain, and often terrifying, exploration of the self that transforms the hero. It's common for budding heroes, whether masculine or feminine,[5] to experience disappointments that call them to their next adventure. A relationship may disintegrate, a job may be lost, or the death of a loved one may devastate. Whatever the precipitating event, it forces reluctant heroes to leave behind all that they know for a quest into unfamiliar territory.

The Call to a Relational Adventure

The three of us were called to our collaborative adventure each in our own way. Susan's call came from a disappointment experienced in her reaching out to a like-minded colleague:

> I work at an institution known for its research related to rural health care, and most of my faculty colleagues conduct research in this topic area. I am the sole person engaged in work related to incivility in nursing education. Thus, I stand alone in terms of others who share my passion locally. After completing my doctorate and joining the tenure track faculty in 2003, I was strongly encouraged to seek out and form collaborative relationships with others across the country who were also interested in incivility. Unfortunately, inexperienced as a scholar in general and not really knowing how to negotiate or forge such a collaboration, my first attempt to

work with someone with a similar interest was, in retrospect, ill-advised. Although we were both willing and interested, neither of us could articulate our specific needs or what we hoped to gain from the relationship. Ultimately, I think we were trying to force a match between similar but different interests and we were never able to determine just exactly where we wanted to go or what we wanted to accomplish. Although well-intentioned, we delved prematurely into a long-distance project that was not well-articulated. Consequently, although I liked the other individual personally, the experience was burdensome and unfulfilling. In the end, the collaboration attempt fizzled. Thus, I was hesitant to enter into another "collaborative relationship" of any kind.

Susan's is an all too common story. Without discussing hopes and dreams or negotiating a contractual agreement at the outset, most hoped-for relationships fizzle, leaving would-be collaborators feeling tentative about future involvements with colleagues.

Allies Arrive on the Scene

"At some point during the distress or confusion of the initial stage, a force or ally intervenes which reinforces, encourages and empowers the hero" (p. 9).[5] Susan describes meeting an ally who helped her break through her reticence:

Unexpectedly, my dissertation resulted in a small buzz in no small part because it turned out that I was not the only one interested in this topic. As luck would have it, however, I may have been the first to get to the finish line with some initial research. One day I received an e-mail from a doctoral student, Cindy Clark, who wanted to discuss my research with me. In a quick click of the send button, we had set a meeting time and before I knew it we were chatting on the phone about incivility. I immediately liked Cindy, not because she was validating my work, but because of her infectious energy. It literally oozed through the phone line. Additionally, she was clearly an intelligent thinker and impassioned about the same topic as I was. Although my MSU colleagues were encouraging and supportive, none of them had ever really "got" what it was about incivility that stirred my passion. Prior to my conversation with Cindy, I had never been able to share a moment of simultaneous enthusiasm about this topic with another person.

Being contacted by Cindy, a kindred spirit who shared Susan's passion and experience with researching academic incivility, was both a boon and a boost. Susan describes how Cindy's risk to reach out melted her hesitation:

> I was also so intrigued that Cindy would actually contact me as the author of a study. This was not because I held myself up on some high horse. Quite the contrary. Rather, my doctoral advisor had implored me to contact authors of studies I had read and assured me it was appropriate to do so. However, I could never quite get around my own inhibitions and actually make a solid contact. It felt too presumptuous on my part. That Cindy either didn't have those inhibitions or chose to be unencumbered by them was intriguing to me. I knew I could learn a lot from this woman!

Cindy writes how participating on an "incivility panel" ignited a mutual attraction that drew her and Kathy together:

> During the summer of 2005, good fortune smiled on me. I was part of a plenary panel selected to present at the 2005 NLN Summit scheduled for the following fall. To prepare for the Summit, the six panel members collaborated via teleconference. During the first conference call, I 'met' Dr. Kathy Heinrich. I was grabbed—hook, line, and sinker. I knew that I really wanted to meet her. So, I called her; we talked for two hours and began corresponding regularly by e-mail and telephone. I could hardly wait to meet her in person at the Summit. With a bit of Idaho in hand (a small gift I brought with me to Baltimore) I met Kathy. I knew immediately who she was—and I hugged her like a *sister*. It was a magical moment—and a portending of what was to come.

For Kathy, meeting Cindy was, ". . . such a shot in the arm, because here was a colleague and a scholar and, now a friend, who energized me with her passion for life and for this topic. Every time I see Cindy's bit of Idaho on our coffee table, it reminds me of our bond."

Our only sadness was Susan's not being at the conference and on the panel, so Cindy arranged for the three of us to speak by phone. Our first conversation was such a warm and intellectually stimulating interchange about topics we rarely discussed with other colleagues that we agreed to speak again in a month. These monthly phone calls continue to this day. For the first year or so, Kathy's ambivalence kept her on the fence:

> To be honest, I'd had enough personal experiences with mean faculty games to last me a lifetime. I didn't want to wallow in those memories by studying incivility; I wanted to help faculty groups get past the mean game playing by giving them the tools to present and publish. So when I was invited to speak about faculty–faculty incivility on the panel where Cindy and I met, I saw it as a brief detour. I figured I'd ask the nurse educator audience to share their free-writes about a time when they felt dismissed or disrespected by a colleague or administrator. After analyzing their stories, I'd work smart by writing a quickie article and get back on track with my consulting and writing *Dare to Share*.

> The more of those monthly phone sessions we had, the more confused I felt. I liked Cindy and Susan so much and found our telephone sessions so invigorating that I wanted to stay connected. I just didn't want to get any more involved with this incivility stuff. So after every conversation, I'd tell myself to bail and let those two go on without me. Then we'd talk again and I'd pencil in the date for our next conference call.

> During one of our monthly phone calls, I found myself saying that I thought our relationship was too special to risk. When I asked Cindy and Susan if they were willing to make wish lists, discuss our fears and concerns, and negotiate a contract, I wondered what I was doing. From the moment they agreed, I knew we were committing to our relationship in a deeper way.

Our Initiation

Initiations usher in a time of testing when the hero is given tasks to perform in the face of obstacles—or dragons—that seem insurmountable.[4,5] Our initiation began with our giving a name to our support circle. This wasn't hard. Our sessions were so energizing that we'd written each other grateful e-mails about our "cosmic connection." Cindy recalls what it was like for her to prepare for our contracting sessions:

> I can still remember with extreme clarity the feelings and thoughts I experienced while generating our "wish lists" and then declaring them openly and unabashedly to one another. Kathy had asked us to work individually on our lists so that we could share them as a group in an upcoming phone call. Crafting my wish list was fairly straightforward. It wasn't the first time I had dreamed about what a scholarly list of desires might include. But holy moley (as Susan would say), it would be the first time I ever said them out loud to myself—much less to others. That part of the process took my breath away.

After all was said and done, this is what our combined wish list looked like:

1. Support team with whom to share joys and sorrows
2. Peer editors
3. Peer mentors
4. Collaborative presentations
5. Co-authored publications
6. Collaborative research

As Cindy soon found out, sharing our wish list was the easy part:

> But what really completely freaked me out was writing down my fears and concerns—and then sharing them honestly and freely with Kathy and Susan. For me, it was speaking the unspeakable. Surely they didn't expect me to dig deeply into my soul and reveal what lay there protected by my own refusal to share what I feared about working together in intimate relationships. I wondered about what might happen if I held back—would Kathy and Susan sense my resistance to exposing my fears and misgivings. Of course they would—I

knew for certain that to be truly engaged in the Cosmic Connection, I needed to be completely authentic. It felt a bit akin to my days in parochial school of entering the confessional. So I prepared and reviewed my lists, then waited for the day when we would exchange them with one another. The phone call began in the usual way—checking in with one another, inquiring about our lives and loves and then getting down to business. Kathy opened the dialogue in her usual eloquent and sensitive way. At first, the phone lines connecting Montana, Idaho, and Connecticut lay silent. It is my only recollection of the Cosmic Connection having little or nothing to say. Usually, the chatter is vibrant and incessant. But that day, it was eerily quiet. Then, very slowly, we shared our dreams, ambitions, hopes, and fears. It was an amazing experience, gentle, soft, cathartic, and straight from the heart. With honest conversation came profound discovery. We learned a lot about ourselves that day—and about each other. As we delicately revealed our fears, we learned that being genuine and 'real' is central and vital to the existence of the Cosmic Connection.

After all the dead space and hesitation and tender sharings, our wishes and concerns generated a list of "we want tos":

1. Maintain our own areas of concentration in the field of incivility.
2. Attribute credit for scholarly work fairly.
3. Put a process in place for negotiating conflict.
4. Make our threesome "safe."
5. Avoid over-politeness so issues won't go unresolved.
6. Ask too much of each other *never.*

To our mutual delight, our next phone session was as chatty as usual with the added benefit of a new-found closeness that came from sharing our fears and concerns.

Now we were ready to negotiate our contract. We committed to keeping our Cosmic Connection zestful by:

1. Assuming best intentions always.
2. Speaking our truth no matter how difficult in a candid, forthright, sensitive manner.

3. Standing for the integrity of our work.
4. Extending invitations that allow for other(s) to say no or yes.

We had no idea at the time how much our contract would serve as a touchstone and centering device each time we met a new obstacle or faced another dragon.

The final step was creating a vision for our partnership. Weaving our ideas together, our vision reads, "Our relationship fuels each partner's passion for her own scholarly endeavors in ways that catalyze her scholarly productivity and enhance her individual and our collective scholarly development." We added this addendum, "This vision for our partnership and contract is a work-in-progress."

Armed with our wish list, contract, and vision, we were as ready as we could be for the tests that lay ahead.

The Bone-Honesty Test

As the coordinator for the Mosby conference, Cindy asked Kathy if she'd like to co-facilitate a workshop session. Kathy tells how this opportunity became a test:

> It takes breaking a good habit to remember why it's important. When Cindy asked me to co-facilitate a workshop on incivility, we were both so excited that we never explored questions like what does each of us want to get from co-presenting; what do we expect from one another as co-presenters; and what's our preferred style for designing a presentation like this one? Nor did we make a contract for our new, co-presenting relationship.
>
> Looking back, it's no wonder we ended up feeling frustrated after two sessions. With a four-hour presentation to design in less than a month, we were stymied. We could be overly polite to avoid conflict or we could, as our contract specified, speak our truth no matter how difficult in a candid, forthright, sensitive manner. Each of us knew what we had to do.

As Kathy recalls:

> In the beginning of our third session, we agreed that we'd both been feeling the tension. I admitted that the disconnect in our relationship was bringing up memories of feeling

betrayed in previous relationships when colleagues wanted credit or took credit for my work. In turn, Cindy shared how her impostor had been called out when she felt that I was expecting her to present just like me. Once I knew that Cindy wanted to carry her weight and she knew that I wanted her to present in her own amazing style, our trust in each other was restored.

Once we cleared up our misunderstandings and misperceptions, it took less than an hour to design our four-hour workshop. Our first task was dividing the workshop into sections that were Cindy's, mine, and both of ours. We'd never done this before in negotiating co-presenting relationships and it worked like a charm.

Once these "yours, mine, and ours" areas were clarified, Kathy recounts how we addressed the differences in our styles:

As we talked it became apparent that Cindy likes to be spontaneous and go in with a general idea of what she's going to talk about and play to her audience. While I like to be spontaneous, I also like to have an outline and know the areas I'm responsible for and what time is allotted for each of my sections. Once we'd figured out our similarities and differences, we were able to proceed with designing our presentation. Only this time instead of a tug of war, we became collaborators. At each juncture, I checked in with Cindy to ensure there was enough openness for her to be spontaneous and Cindy made sure that I felt that we had enough structure.

Over-politeness and avoidance would have gotten us nowhere, whereas facing our differences with what Cindy calls "bone-honesty" made for a respectful collaboration. It turns out that these "yours, mine, and ours" conversations continue to make all the difference in our collaborative endeavors.

The Rock Star Test

The next test came dressed in an unusual disguise—success. Although nurses are gifted at supporting each other when one of us is down and out, we have little experience with handling our feelings of envy and competition when a colleague is successful.[1] Because in the past the price tag for success for women has been going it alone,[1] many nurses stay quiet and hide their successes to keep collegial relationships intact. Susan's story goes like this:

> Recently I provided a workshop in a national venue that went better than expected. I spoke to a standing-room-only crowd and the topic hit a chord. Subsequently, follow-up opportunities resulted in my name getting public air time in some nursing education circles. I'd done an NLN audio-Web seminar and had several publications come out around this same time. Thus, my name was suddenly visible in multiple venues. In addition, incivility is a hot topic. Many graduate students appear to be interested in studying various aspects of the incivility topic. On several occasions I've had people actually tell me they have read everything that I've written. One lady told me it was an honor to meet me and joked that she felt like asking for my autograph. Another said she couldn't wait to get back to her colleagues and tell them she met me.
>
> I joked one day to Kathy and Cindy that to be the focus of this level of professional admiration, much of which seems unfounded, made me feel like a rock star. One thing I was unprepared for was the surreal nature of the "fame" that accompanies professional successes.

Susan is fortunate in having a supportive group of colleagues at work who celebrate her successes with flowers and her beloved M&M's. Our Cosmic Connection supports her in other ways:

> I'm grateful to have my cosmic sisters to help me work through this. The first thing I get from them is support. They allow me to talk through strategic questions I have about how to handle various interactions and the most appropriate next steps to achieve my career goals. For example, they help me work through issues regarding the value of what I offer and how to charge fees that reflect that value for workshops and consultations. However, they do more than that. Although I've been in situations where I'm meeting someone of great

significance for me and have been awestruck, I find being the center of this type of adulation a bit disconcerting and humbling. My "sisters" help me to recognize my affliction and work through the various manifestations of "imposter syndrome" by validating and reminding me of what I have contributed to the field. There is nothing ingratiating about the way they do so. Rather, it is a practical, matter-of-fact approach, removed of just enough emotion to allow me to examine my work and contributions objectively.

Susan's sharing her success allows her to overcome her impostor feelings surrounded by a support circle of work colleagues and cosmic sisters.

The Trifecta Test

In our wish list, we'd written that we want to present as a threesome. Cindy calls this "The Trifecta." Kathy was contacted by a school that wanted a day-long faculty development workshop on cultivating civility. Although we recommended the Trifecta, the school was leaning toward hiring two out of the three of us. How would we decide which two it would be? Cindy tells it this way:

> What might have been a deal-breaker for other groups became a transformative experience for the Cosmic Connection. We agreed from the start that Kathy would present no matter what. She was the person first contacted by the school and she brings the expertise in faculty–faculty incivility. How would Susan and I feel if only one of us were selected? All three of us agreed that it was a professional, not a personal, matter. That being the case we knew we needed to do something intentional to develop an impartial proposal.
>
> Writing this proposal brought us face to face with the areas of overlap in Cindy's and Susan's research on incivility. To clarify this overlap meant having another "yours, mine, and ours" discussion in which each of us identified the something special we bring to workshop presentations. Meanwhile, Cindy came up with a brilliant solution to depersonalize the hiring process. As a result, our proposals now include a three-presenter option

along with two, two-presenter options. All three options describe the theoretical content to be offered with no names attached. When schools select their desired option, they are choosing the presenters as well. So whether it's the trifecta or some combination of two of us presenting, it's all good.

Cindy sums it up this way:

> What could have been fraught with conflict and disagreement was liberating and enlightening. We are stronger for it. I fully believe that the three of us are each other's biggest, baddest cheerleaders. It's fun taking turns lifting each other up on the proverbial pedestal and loving every minute of it.

Conclusion

In the final stage of transformation, the hero must return to the world with some gift to help restore the community.[6] Although our Cosmic Connection is still in the initiation phase, every so often we catch a glimmer of the gift we will share with the nursing community. We used to think it would be the insights from our incivility research. After co-authoring this chapter, we're beginning to suspect our gift has more to do with living out civility in our zestful collegial partnerships. We hope that sharing our challenges has given you the courage, along with a few strategies, to explore this new relational territory alongside us.

TIP

Keep collegial partnerships zestful by negotiating what's yours, mine, and ours.

References

1. Eichenbaum, L., & Orbach, S. (1988). *Between women: Love, envy, and competition in women's friendships.* Scranton, PA: Haddon Craftsmen.
2. Higher Education Research Institute. (1996). *A social change model for leadership development* (Version III). Los Angeles: Regents of the University of California.

3. Emry, R. A., & Holmes, O. (2005, Spring). Civility: The value of valuing differences. *Senate Forum, XX*(2), 3–6. Retrieved September 12, 2007, from: http://www.fullerton.edu/senate/forum/Spring_2005.pdf
4. Campbell, J. (1988). *The power of myth*. New York: Doubleday.
5. Noble, K. (1994). *The sound of the silver horn: Reclaiming heroism in contemporary women's lives*. Boston: Shambala Press.
6. Noble, K. D. (1990). The female hero: A quest for healing and wholeness. *Women and Therapy, 9*(4), 3–18.

How Expressing Wishes and Concerns Keeps Collaborations Zestful

89

Human life is the most difficult classroom until you learn the simple fact that your truth is your power, your salvation, your fulfillment, your purpose, and your way. Once you can truly believe that, life becomes the joyous and abundant garden that it is meant to be.

Emmanuel

If you want a zestful collaboration, admit your fears and concerns about working together at the outset. Sounds paradoxical, doesn't it? In that past, I'd always kept my misgivings to myself, because I thought I might turn off a potential collaborator by expressing any doubts. In fact, the Cosmic Connection was the first partnership I'd been in where we verbalized our concerns as well as our wishes; where our contract/covenant took our concerns into account, leaving us feeling safe to proceed. Even with all this, you read how scary it was for Cindy and me to be bone-honest with each other as co-presenters. At first it took every shred of courage we had to face dragons as they stomped into our relational field; I'm happy to report that it gets easier with each dragon met and test passed. Consciousness must be a contagion, because I'm finding myself becoming more candid in other collaborative relationships.

Although it may be counterintuitive to raise concerns at the outset, when such discussions are left until after problems have interfered with the task, it may be too late. So don't wait! Take a moment to consider your fears or concerns related to a collaborative undertaking with a colleague–friend (Jot Box 89-1).

Jot Box 89-1

Your fears and concerns about collaborating are:

_____

_____

_____

_____

_____

_____

_____

How was that for you? If thinking about your fears and concerns made you feel a bit anxious, you're not alone. Instead of admitting that relationships are as unpredictable as the ocean tides, that communications can tangle like seaweed on the rocks despite the best of intentions, as nurses we tend to close our eyes and dive into relational pools without water wings, never mind life preservers. It's the rare presenting–publishing project in which relationships with collaborators aren't tested in some way. Therefore, it's more realistic to assume that in the course of any creative endeavor stresses, misunderstandings and disagreements are all part of the process.

Prevention being the better part of cure, there are three steps that keep communications mindful and collaborations conscious:

1. Know that your creative collaborations will be tested.
2. Share fears and concerns right after wish lists.
3. Write contract/covenants in ways that allow concerns as well as wishes to be acknowledged and addressed.

Then you'll be able to swim with, through, and around any currents and undertows that arise secure in knowing that they'll never reach tsunami size or force.

TIP

It's easier to express your fears and concerns, difficult as it may be, now rather than waiting for your first misunderstanding.

Conclusion: Commit to Cultivating Support Circles

90

> *What, exactly is "mind-ful-ness"? Mindfulness is the direct, immediate, and vivid experience of whatever is arising here and now. It is a nonjudgmental awareness that does not get caught up in thoughts or concepts or "stories" of any kind. It is sometimes called "bare attention." Mindfulness is simply knowing and experiencing just as it is.*

Stephen Cope

The constant in the stories you have just read about creative collaborations is how mindful communication helps partners maximize the joys and negotiate the challenges involved in peer-mentoring, peer-editing, and partnership relationships. Keeping zest scores as high as eye-glitter scores is a matter of writing concerns into covenants and addressing wishes in contracts. Then, with your support circle rooting for you all the way, there's no dare to share that will be too big or too scary to tackle.

Your Nurse–Companions

As their free-writes reflect, your companions are considering partnership possibilities and creative collaborations. Each responded to the following question: "What's your next step in cultivating a support circle?"

Keri wrote:

> Before I ever read this section, I'd been communicating online with a nurse practitioner who's also practicing on the reservation where she grew up. After reading about peer editing and peer mentoring, I wrote her an "Ask" e-mail about setting up a phone session to explore the possibility of establishing an "official partnership" to support each other's presenting and publishing. And who knows, maybe we'll even figure out some other ways to collaborate.

Betty's free-write reads:

> I'm between dare-to-share projects, so I've scheduled a session with a peer mentor at my favorite café to brainstorm ideas for my next project. As we talk, I'm betting we'll come up with a work-smart project that we can do together.

Justin wrote:

> I'm pretty psyched because our group just got our paper accepted to make a presentation at the "Association of Male Nurses" regional conference this summer and I hope to connect with potential colleague–friends and maybe even a potential mentor or two, while I'm there.

Although Keri is the companion who's had the greatest epiphany about cultivating support circles, Betty and Justin both have plans for expanding their support circles. Before you see where you are with the same question your companions just answered, review the "15 Powerful Practices for Cultivating a Support Circle":[1]

1. Draw your support circle.
2. Choose to collaborate with colleague–friends.
3. Create opportunities to expand your support circle by reaching out.

4. Commit to setting aside the time and energy for a dare-to-share project.
5. Compose a wish list that makes your eyes glitter.
6. Discern and dialogue about what's yours, mine, and ours.
7. Consider fears and concerns about collaborating.
8. Contract in ways that honor wishes and protect vulnerabilities.
9. Carve out a work-smart sequence by turning co-presenters into co-authors.
10. Check to see if your collaborations pass the zest test.
11. Communicate mindfully to keep your collaboration vibrant.
12. Close the presentation phase before initiating the publication phase.
13. Convey gratitude for your collaborator(s') gifts and contributions.
14. Congratulate yourselves on breaking trail in relational territory.
15. Celebrate accomplishments.

Now it's your turn to respond to the free-write question in Jot Box 90-1.

Jot Box 90-1

What's your next step in cultivating a support circle?

_____

_____

_____

_____

_____

You may be wondering what life will be like as you take dares to share by reaching out to your ever-expanding circle of colleague–friends. The next section shows and tells what it's like to live the dare-to-share lifestyle before sending you off on your next adventure.

TIP

Commit to cultivating a support circle one colleague–friend at a time.

Reference

1. Heinrich, K. T., et al. (2003). From partners to passionate scholars: Preparing nurse educators for the new millennium. *Annual Review of Nursing Education, 1,* 129–130.

Small Steps:
Send Off

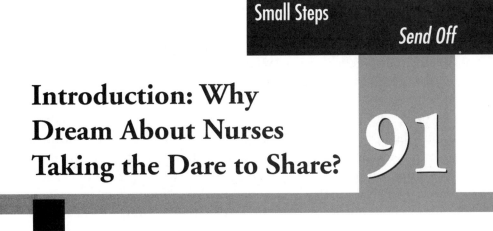

Introduction: Why Dream About Nurses Taking the Dare to Share?

91

You may say I'm a dreamer,
but I'm not the only one.

John Lennon

I wrote *Dare to Share* because I've noticed something remarkable. Sharing what they do makes nurses' eyes glitter. At a time when many "in education, practice, research, and community settings are disillusioned and depressed about the current state of nursing, rather than inspired and hopeful about our profession" (p. 24),[1] nurses who present and publish are a vibrant exception. This is true regardless of their specialty area, years in practice, work setting, or working conditions. And, whether they have an R.N. or a doctorate, whether they publish in *Nursing Spectrum* or *Nursing Research*, to a one, they use words like "delighted," "thrilled," and "exhilarated" to describe how they feel when they present and publish.

This observation got me to dreaming. I imagine what it's going to be like when *all* nurses in school are taught to present and publish by support circles of educators and student colleagues. A time when, after graduation, nurses expand their support circles to include professional colleagues, all of whom dare to share. I envision a time when their presentation-turned-publication projects co-create a literature

403

written in a variety of styles that speak to nurses at all educational levels in all practice arenas. When these circles of passionate nurses create zestful workplaces with zero tolerance for competitive, joy-stealing games; and when these zestful workplaces attract the best and the brightest into nursing and nursing education as a career choice. A time when, with no more need to recruit clinicians or educators, resources are freed up to develop nurses' ability to share what they do in venues and in vehicles that engage lay as well as professional audiences. As I read articles by visionaries who call for *all* nurses to contribute to our knowledge base in the new millennium,[2,3] I knew I was not the only one weaving such daydreams. If a glitter in the eyes of individual nurses can revitalize an entire profession, then preparing nurses to share what they do is a vision worth manifesting.

Your Nurse–Companions

When I asked your nurse–companions this question, "Would you like to read about an RN who dares to share on a daily basis?", their free-write responses were a unanimous "yes."

> Keri wrote:
>
> Now that I am in the process of writing a manuscript and have a practitioner–colleague in my support circle, I'm really interested in hearing from a nurse whose life is a dare to share.
>
> Betty wrote:
>
> Yes, I would very much like to read the story of a nurse who dares to share as an everyday occurrence. I'm hoping for some pointers on how to integrate dares to share into my day-to-day life as well as my practice.
>
> Justin wrote:
>
> Sure!

If, like your companions, you want to learn from a nurse who is vibrant with sharing what she does, then the storytelling chapter that comes next will more than satisfy.

There's no nurse I know whose eyes glitter more than Irene O'Day's. On any given day, you'd be lucky to catch her digging the dandelions from her garden after she's written a letter to the editor of *The Hartford Courant* and sent e-mails to senators and congressmen expressing her concerns before her afternoon presentation at the men's prison and her evening meeting with her women's political action group. In this final section, Irene's storytelling chapter shows you how life can unfurl for nurses who dare to share. After talking about the glow that comes from being in the flow of sharing, there's a "send off" message for you encrypted into the Coda.

References

1. Pesut, D. (2004). Creating the future through renewal: 2003–2005 presidential call to action. *Reflections on Nursing Leadership, 30*(1), 24.
2. Bunkers, S. S. (2000). The nurse scholar of the 21st century. *Nursing Science Quarterly, 13*(2), 116–123.
3. Riley, J. M., Beal, J., Levi, P., & McCauseland, M. P. (2002). Revisioning nursing scholarship. *Journal of Nursing Scholarship, 34*(4), 383–389.

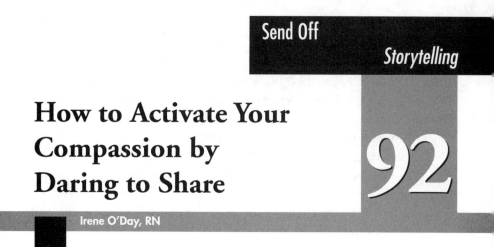

How to Activate Your Compassion by Daring to Share

92

Irene O'Day, RN

> *Compassion enjoins us to respond to pain, and wisdom guides the skillfulness of the response, telling us when and how to respond. Through compassion our lives become an expression of all that we understand, care about and value.*
>
> Sharon Salzberg

I'm a 78-year-old retired nurse, wife, mother of four, and grandmother of three. For someone who lives life fast forward, writing this chapter has been a revelation. Looking back on my life, I've discovered that at each step along the way, there's been a meaningful turning point that's become a call to compassion. The word *compassion, com* ("with") and *passion* ("suffer"), literally means to share the pain of another. While I've long known that nursing allowed me to share the pain of others, retirement is giving me the freedom to respond to calls to compassion in new and unexpected ways, many of which involve a dare to share.

During an interview with Joseph Campbell, Bill Moyers asked, "How will we know if we are on the right path?" Campbell's reply was, in effect, we will know when, in moments of synchronicity, we come across just the right book or in a chance encounter a guide appears to point the way, or one door closes and another opens.[1] In this chapter I tell about the paths that nursing has opened up for me, and the synchronicities that confirm the rightness of this path, to encourage you to share your own experiences. For when you do, the lives that you touch with your presentations and your writings, the people you meet, and the opportunities that open up to you will be as rewarding as the best days of your nursing career.

Nightingale's Life Calls Me to Nursing

An early school assignment led me to read about the life of Florence Nightingale for a book report. I still recall the intense feelings her story evoked in me at that impressionable age. Nightingale felt her call to minister to the sick was divinely inspired, named it her "must," and believed that it sustained her throughout the difficulties in her life. After reading this book, I knew without a doubt that I wanted to be a nurse. While in high school, my call to nursing was affirmed when I began volunteering at the local hospital. Within a short time I was hired as a "ward aide" and allowed to perform some patient care, which I loved doing.

These experiences helped qualify me for admission to the Hartford Hospital School of Nursing. Established in 1877, this was the fourth school to be organized under the Florence Nightingale plan for training nurses. Linda Rogers, an early superintendent and a former student of Nightingale's, incorporated Nightingale's philosophy that nursing is an art that requires "as exclusive a devotion, as hard a preparation as any painter's or sculptor's work"[2] into our curriculum. Our first course was called "Nursing Arts," where, along with basic skills, I learned the importance of seeing the whole person in patients.

A call to act came during my second year when another classmate and I decided to circulate a petition to improve our Diet Kitchen (D.K.) assignment. Instead of learning about special diets, students spent most of their time scrubbing pots and mopping floors. When we submitted our petition to the school administration, we knew we were risking dismissal, remember this was 1949. Instead we were praised for our "Nightingale like" action and the curriculum was changed. How's that for a dare to share?

Life as a Practicing Nurse

After graduation, at a time when patients were separated by gender, I worked as a staff nurse and later as head nurse on a post-surgical, male unit. During those years, I was selected to be an assistant clinical instructor at my school of nursing and I was pleased to be able to pass on our history and traditions to new students. I left nursing after I married to raise four children and jumped back into uniform occasionally to care for family members who were hospitalized. As the children grew, I took a part-time position in a local public health agency that included home health and school nursing, where the flexible hours allowed me to keep up with my children's schedules.

Throughout my career I stayed up-to-date by attending classes, meetings, seminars, conferences, and conventions in whatever my nursing interest was at the time. Whether it was surgery, public health, school nursing, vocational education, or home hospice, I found that the presentations were always the same: lecture, a few visual aids, and lots of handouts. After about 20 minutes, with eyes glazed over I stopped concentrating and mentally drifted off or doodled. I'd leave the class on overload, retain only a portion of the information, and rarely read the handouts. If a short quiz was required for CEUs, I couldn't be sure of my answers.

When it came time for me to teach, I taught as I was taught, knowing no other way. Until I enrolled in a college certification program to teach secondary school health and vocational education. There I learned a new approach for presenting content and skills called P.P.P.T.—Preparation, Presentation, Practice, Test—that engaged the students as much as possible in the presentation and reduced the content to the most basic interpretation and understanding. Another dare to share came with being hired to develop and teach a Nurse's Aide program in a high school. Because there were no established guidelines, I was asked, along with other instructors, to write a teacher's manual for this program to be used statewide. That was my first experience with writing and being published, and a thrilling one at that.

Retirement Opens New Pathways

As I neared retirement, I began attending programs for my own spiritual growth at a retreat center run by the Sisters of Mercy. Gradually, I was asked to assist the nuns who were beginning to offer programs with a physical focus. By this time I had interned with Bernie Siegel,[1] I was teaching Therapeutic Touch, and had joined the Nurse-Healers Professional Association and the American Holistic Nurses Association

(AHNA). Both organizations were attempting to reconnect nurses with the art of nursing that I feared had been lost forever. As a member, I learned about energy medicine, guided imagery, healing music, and other integrative modalities. I'd also made an in-depth study of the life of a 12th-century mystic, Hildegard of Bingen, who is considered a healer in the early history of nursing. So when the Mercy Center directors asked me to share all of this, I felt like I had come home.

I was concerned that the calls to compassion would cease with retirement, but, if anything, the calls increased. Soon after I retired, as a volunteer with the Lung Association, I was asked to give testimony at a hearing at our State Capitol in favor of an act to prohibit smoking in public places and in places of employment. I wrote my speech, submitted 75 copies, and gave my testimony about secondhand smoke being preventable beginning with these words, "As a registered nurse of more than 40 years of experience, I have seen first hand the damage done to my patients by tobacco smoke. I speak for all those who choose not to smoke . . . infants and small children, pregnant women" and citing the research that supported my clinical observations. It was one of the most stressful things I'd ever done, but the elation I felt when the bill was finally enacted was worth every minute of the impostor fears and stage fright I'd endured.

Nightingale Reappears with a New Call

Several years later, I attended a ceremony on August 12, 2001, at the National Cathedral in Washington, DC, commemorating the inclusion of Florence Nightingale in the Episcopal Church calendar of Lesser Feasts and Fasts. After spending time in England researching Nightingale's writings, Barbara Dossey and her nursing colleagues convinced Church officials that Nightingale met the criteria for an honor wrongfully denied her by the Church of England. I was thrilled beyond measure to attend this historic moment in nursing. Many top dignitaries in government and nursing were there along with many nurses. Some of us were in tears as Dossey delivered the keynote address, in which she said:

> A part of Nightingale's wisdom lies in each of us. She would be at home in our world. I imagine hearing her voice as she tells each of us to identify our "must" and to fight for a healthcare system driven by the needs of patients. She would

encourage each of us collectively to join together to actualize our visions. She would ask us if we are documenting through research our work and services. Nightingale, the master networker, would want us always to know who is in charge, who our representatives and senators are. She would ask us to educate and inform them through research findings, so they can develop legislation for healthcare reform that makes sense.[3]

Hearing Dossey's words transformed me. I knew then and there what direction my life should take and ever since opportunities to learn, to speak, and to write that I never dreamed possible continue to arise.

Retreats

By now, Sr. Pat had become my mentor and eventually my spiritual director. Together we conducted retreats for student nurses and later I presented programs on my own. Because I felt it was so urgently needed, I offered to conduct a retreat for nurses entitled "A Celebration of Nursing." Held on May 12, Nightingale's birthday, this day-long workshop opened with a guided-imagery session in which Nightingale welcomed participants and urged them to use this time for self-healing. After a meditation, they dialogued about their call to nursing. At noon, we gathered around a lit candle to celebrate the "Nightingale Moment," a ritual observed annually by nurses around the world in honor of our foundress. A poem written by a nurse was read, and the morning concluded with a recitation of the Nightingale pledge. After lunch, walking the beach and circling the labyrinth allowed time for more reflection. The day ended with a symbolic hand-washing ritual and the saying of a blessing that each nurse bestowed on another:

> May the God of Compassion be with you, holding you close when you are weary and hurt and alone, and when there is rain in your heart. And may you be warm eyes of Compassion for your friends when they reach out to you in need. May the blessing of Compassion be upon you.

Always a moving experience for me, participants' comments on evaluations confirmed that this was a day of healing for them. So when the AHNA asked for feedback about how the "Nightingale Moment" was observed, I sent in my report, which was published in a newsletter along with similar observances. I continued to offer this nurses retreat for several years and then passed it on to another holistic nurse.

In time, Sr. Pat invited me to become a lay Associate of the Sisters of Mercy. As such, I joined in covenant with the Mercy mission of reaching out to the underserved, the marginalized, and especially to women and children. When Sr. Pat became a chaplain at the state prisons for men and women, she invited me to join her in this ministry by becoming a prison volunteer. I readily agreed. When I was asked to develop a program using meditation for stress management and to incorporate some of the holistic practices I'd learned, Sr. Pat advised me to, "Keep it short, simple, and varied." She cautioned me that some of the inmates might have limited education, short attention span, language barriers, and brain damage due to drug abuse. I assured her that nurses handle such challenges all the time.

The program I developed was based on Herbert Benson's Relaxation Response and included progressive relaxation, guided imagery, music for the Mozart effect, and centering prayer. Translating the theory behind these practices, so the men would understand the physiology of stress and be more willing to participate, was my greatest challenge. My engineer son taught me some "gear-head" terms, and my ex–GI husband peer mentored my presentations. This male feedback was invaluable, as were Sr. Pat's ongoing suggestions. The men were hesitant at first, then after we introduced ourselves they relaxed, became focused on the content, and bonded with one another.

Using techniques learned in retreat work to engage them in sharing, at the end of the eight-week session their evaluations affirmed that most of my objectives were met. I was thrilled when on the last day one man presented me with a poster he had drawn of a man's head with all of the parts involved in the stress-and-relaxation response properly labeled. He then described the entire process using all the correct words. It was then I knew Sr. Pat had been right all along.

Nurse Colleagues Call Me to Dare to Share

I continue to offer programs at the prison and consider myself blessed to be able to do so at my age. When I noticed Patricia Winstead-Fry's call for nurses to submit stories of unusual nursing experiences for a book she was writing, I submitted a story about my prison experiences. To my surprise and delight, it was published in her book *Ordinary Miracles in Nursing*.[4] I was especially pleased, because I wanted older nurses to know that we can still feel as fulfilled, if not more, in retirement.

I contacted Ginette Ferszt after reading an article in *Advance for Nurses* about a program that she and another nurse had developed for helping prisoners cope with grief. After Ginette kindly sent me pamphlets they'd written for their program along with encouraging words,[5] I developed a program for my inmates that begins with them reading the pamphlet aloud followed by sharing their feelings about the losses in their lives. They are then asked to think about someone they had lost, and what they would like to say to that person or persons, if they had the opportunity. I invite them to free-write about their reflections. Beyond assuring them that no one would read them, I promise to take their free-writes home and in a ceremony in my garden I burn them and bury the ashes around a beautiful rose bush. As a final healing measure, I play a guided imagery tape by Belleruth Naparastek titled *Ease Grief,* which contains soothing messages for healing the pain of loss.[6] I've presented this program several times, and I continue to get requests for more sessions and more tapes.

Life as an Activist

I've taken to calling myself a kitchen activist, because I don't even have to leave home to work for change. The calls to compassion that began with the ring of my kitchen phone are just as likely to appear as e-mails these days. A short time ago, I met with a highly motivated group of women to charter a local branch of a federation of a women's political organization. Being involved with this group and encouraged by the activism of the Sisters of Mercy, I am drawn to speak out on issues of health care for women and children, the war, and other social concerns. I now have time to write letters to the editor, some of which have been published, and to attend rallies and speak to groups to promote positive change.

The Internet makes this incredibly easy. By signing up for action alerts at the Web sites of the ANA political action link, the Nightingale Initiative for Global Health, the Physicians for Social Responsibility, the Sisters of Mercy Justice link, as well as those of peace and environmental organizations, I can sign a petition or e-mail a message to my state and federal lawmakers to ask their support for legislation that addresses my concerns. The term for activism that stems from or connects us to our spirit is *spiritual activism*. In *Urgent Message From Mother*, Jean Shinoda Bolen writes, "There is in all of us a tendency toward the spiritual—an orientation toward an invisible presence, to something greater than ourselves that cannot be fully known. Spirituality unites us—in silence, in awe, in devotion and in soul connections" (p. 12).[7] Soul connections like these move me to participate in causes that resonate with deeply held convictions and beliefs. All of this has given new meaning to my life.

Live Your Passion by Activating Your Compassion

At mid-life, I could not have imagined the life I am now living. As I approach my eighth decade, I can hardly believe that each day still holds so much meaning for me as I continue to "follow my bliss."[1] I have discovered that my calls to compassion, when nurtured by prayer, meditation, inspirational reading, and caring companions, enrich my life beyond measure, and how everything I do for myself and others now becomes heart centered. As it turns out, many of these calls involve speaking and writing. Here are a few suggestions for activating your call to compassion:

- **Tell your story.** So many venues and vehicles are now available for nurses to tell their stories. In fact, I just came across an invitation for nurses to tell their stories in *Advance OnLine*.[8] This is an easy dare to share; go to this Web site and type in your story. Or, write a reflection on your professional life's journey. You'll be amazed at what you'll remember. It wasn't until I pulled out my nursing yearbook in the midst of writing this chapter that I remembered the DKT petition that changed our curriculum.
- **Read inspirational books.** I've included some of my favorites, especially those written by nurses, in the reference list. Sue Monk Kidd, a nurse for many years, felt compelled to become a writer at mid-life. Her book, entitled *When the Heart Waits— Spiritual Direction for Life's Sacred Questions*,[9] holds great meaning for me and will for any nurse who reads it at mid-life. Barbara Dossey's books on Florence Nightingale's life[10,11] are a great inspiration to me as are all books about women who,

when pushed against the tide, overcome their obstacles to reach their dreams.

- **Expand your circle.** Reach out to others from different walks of life. I belong to a circle of women who are involved in many art forms as well as spiritual beliefs. We share our ideas and diverse interests and help each other stretch and grow. You may want to consider joining or starting a book club to share ideas and learn from each other.

- **Bring nursing's history alive.** Interview an older nurse and share her story. I used to love talking with older nurses, especially when they were my patients, because their life experiences were a source of living nursing history. Older nurses, whether they're hang gliding or consulting or volunteering, can serve as models for meaningful retirement.[12]

- **Dream big.** Diane Carlson Evans, a Vietnam War Army nurse, sought funding for a statue at the Vietnam War Memorial in Washington, DC to honor the 265,000 women, mostly nurses, who served so heroically during that war. She proposed the statue as a way to promote healing for the women who were physically and emotionally traumatized by battle. Each Memorial and Veteran's day, nurses and their families gather at the statue to share poems, stories and music they have written to heal themselves and each other.

Conclusion

On behalf of that master networker, Florence Nightingale, I invite you to continue her legacy of boldly speaking out and writing by connecting to the spirit within to bring hope and healing to the world. For when you act on your compassion by daring to share, you'll find yourself on a path that will surprise and delight you in ways you cannot begin to imagine.

References

1. Campbell, J., with Moyers, B. (1988). *The power of myth.* New York: Doubleday.
2. Nightingale, F. (1868, June 1). Una and the Lion. *Good Words,* p. 362.

3. Dossey, B. (2000). Florence Nightingale's message for today. *Beginnings: The Official Newsletter of the American Holistic Nurses' Association, 20*(1), 1–10.
4. Winstead-Fry, P. (2006). *Ordinary miracles in nursing.* Sudbury, MA: Jones and Bartlett Publishers.
5. Ferszt, G., & Taylor, P. (2001). *When death enters your life, a grief pamphlet for people in prisons or jails.* Alexandria, VA: The Grace Project.
6. Naparastek, B. (1992). *Ease grief* (CD). Available at: http://www.health journeys.com
7. Bolen, J. S. (2005). *Urgent message from mother: Gather the women, save the world.* York, ME: Conari Press.
8. *Advance OnLine.* Available at: http://nursing.advanceweb.com/main.aspx
9. Kidd, S. M. (1990). *When the heart waits: Spiritual direction for life's sacred moments.* San Francisco: Harper San Francisco.
10. Dossey, B., Selander, L., & Beck, D. M. (2005). *Florence Nightingale today: Healing, leadership, global action.* Washington, DC: American Nurses Association.
11. Dossey, B. (2000). *Florence Nightingale: Mystic, visionary, healer.* Philadelphia: Lippincott Williams & Wilkins.
12. Chinn, P. L. (2008). Reflections on retirement and related matters. In N. H. Oermann (Ed.), *Annual review of nursing education: Clinical nursing education* (Vol. 6). New York: Springer.

How to Get a Glow from the Flow of Good Work

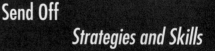

It's not just a job, it's a calling.
It's not for the weak or the faint.
It takes kindness and wit.
And strength that won't quit.
Happy Nurse's Day.

Hartline, Hallmark Card

Irene is an RN with no special degrees or certifications. What she does have is a calling to nursing that's lasted almost 60 years, a hero in Florence Nightingale, a love of learning, a deep compassion for others, a sense of spirituality that informs her actions, a commitment to excellence, and a desire to do good work. Whether she's designing a presentation for her inmates at the prison or writing her *Dare to Share* chapter for us, she's totally focused on her task and exuberant about her latest adventure. Irene's got the glow that comes from being in the flow of doing good work.

Mihaly Csikszentmihalyi[1] who has made a life's study of optimal human experience, has found that almost everyone feels more creative, concentrated, and motivated when involved in an activity requiring skill and patience. Even in adversity, people feel best when they are in the thick of things, while at leisure they often report feeling dull and dissatisfied. He says:

> If you enjoy sticking your neck out and trying to operate at your best or even beyond your best, if you're lucky enough to get that combination, then you're more likely to learn new things, to become better at what you're doing, to invent new things, to discover new things. We seem to be a species that has been blessed by this kind of thirst for pushing the envelope . . . in our nervous system, maybe by chance or at random, an association has been made between pleasure and challenge, or looking for new challenges.[1]

It's this thirst for challenge that moves us into the flow of good work.

While "flow experiences"[1] can happen anytime, from making art to making love, this feeling of total involvement in effortless performance outside of time happens more often in work than in leisure time.[2] Practitioners in a profession experience this flow when society views them as doing "good work." When Irene graduated in 1950, nursing values were more in alignment with societal values, and her story has all six of the characteristics exhibited by such practitioners:[2]

1. Experiences a call to the profession.
2. Sustained by a spiritual tradition.
3. Values competence and character.
4. Lives by an inner set of values and a moral compass.
5. Anchored in the tradition of teachers and mentors from whom she learned.
6. Operates from a clear code of ethics.

Since her student days, Irene has been speaking out against misalignments that threaten the flow of nurses doing good work. For seasoned practitioners like Irene, speaking out about misalignments becomes an opportunity, "to articulate the essence of their calling. To draw the line to indicate what is acceptable and what is not, and to act decisively against individuals and institutions that trespass on it" (p. 219).[2] In so doing, "good ancestors" like Irene stand for excellence and uphold ethical standards in ways that give heart to other practitioners.

One of the symptoms of a profession misaligned with society's values is concern for the fate of that profession.[2] With many disillusioned and fearing for the future of nursing,[3] one way that we as nurses can recover our flow is by daring to share our good work(s). In traveling the country, I am seeing that "when nurses are taught to present and publish, their discontent with jobs and fears for the future of nursing melt. With eyes a'glitter, their relationships become collaborative and their workplaces zestful" (p. 5).[4] If you want to shine with some of Irene's glow, it's as easy and as challenging as daring to share. Your nurse–companions will respond to a question sure to inspire you to consider your next dare-to-share challenge.

Nurse–Companions

When asked, "What topic do you feel passionate enough about to speak up, out, and often?" Here is how your nurse–companions responded.

Keri wrote:

> My experiences with my poster presentation and writing a manuscript helped me to see how my life and my practice are interwoven. I feel passionate enough about native nurse practitioners working with their own people to speak and write about my own, their, and our combined experiences.

Betty wrote:

> I've discovered that my passion is helping staff nurses share all the amazing things they do in presentations and publications.

Justin's free-write says:

> I feel passionate about men in nursing and speaking out to ensure that nurse educators and nursing education are sensitive to their gender, learning styles, and communication styles.

If this question had been posed earlier in *Dare to Share,* your companions might not have been able to summarize their passion so succinctly. By completing the exercises and worksheets, a presentation, and a manuscript, Keri, Betty, and Justin have given words to their passionate focus, and in the process defined their future direction for dares to share. Now that they've learned the small steps and experienced the pains and pleasures related to working smart by presenting and publishing, they're ready to embark on the next leg of their dare-to-share journey. Now it's your turn to answer the same question in Jot Box 93-1.

─────── **Jot Box 93-1** ───────

What do I feel passionate enough about to speak up, out, and often about?

_____

_____

_____

_____

_____

_____

_____

_____

_____

Rereading what you wrote, were you able to:

1. Summarize your passion in one sentence.
2. Define your future direction.
3. Recognize your readiness to embark on your next dare-to-share adventure.

If you answered, "yes," then you're ready to stick your neck out, learn new things, push the envelope, get pleasure from taking new challenges, and in no time at all you'll find you've got the glow from the flow of sharing good work.

References

1. Csikszentmihalyi, M. (1997). _Finding flow._ New York: Basic Books.
2. Gardner, H., Csikszentmihalyi, M., & Damon, W. (2001). _Good work: When excellence and ethics meet._ New York: Basic Books.
3. Pesut, D. (2004). Creating the future through renewal: 2003–2005 presidential call to action. _Reflections on Nursing Leadership, 30_(1), 24.
4. Heinrich, K. T. (2007). Joy-stealing: 10 mean games faculty play and how to stop the gaming. _Nurse Educator, 32_(1), 1–5.

Coda

Be well, do good work, and keep in touch.

Garrison Keillor

Now that our journey is coming to an end, you're ready to set off on the dare-to-share trail. So rather than a conclusion, this is a heartfelt send-off with three homespun reminders.

Be well! Whenever your inner critic tries to make you feel like an impostor, you'll know how to *shift your perspective* to see yourself as creative; *self-reflect* to explore your inner landscape; practice the *strategies and skills* that turn everyday experiences into presentations and publications; and cultivate a *support circle* overflowing with colleague–friends. Doing so will keep the glitter in your eyes.

Do good work! Speak from your truth, engage your audience and your readers with as much passion as compassion, and be prepared. Even as you discover the joys of presenting and publishing, your commitment will be tested. Along the way, you'll meet surprise twists and turns and you may even stumble on occasion. Trust that when you persevere, you'll come to a place where you can see so far into the distance to a vista so breathtaking you'll be filled with an urge to put what you see into words. You'll want others to know that it's worth facing down any dragon to your newfound clarity.

Keep in touch! Stay connected to those colleague–friends who care enough to dare you to share. For it is your peer mentors and peer editors, co-presenters and co-authors, and collaborators and partners who form the circle that supports your efforts—who ask you when you're nearly done, what your plans are for your next adventure, and, oh, by the way, how they can help. Whether it's a hug or tough love that you need, they're there. You'll find that staying in touch with them keeps you in touch with yourself.

It's time! Take to the path, claim who you are, and manifest your vision for nursing, knowing that every time you share what you do, you open that possibility to all of us. *Go well!*

Appendix A.
Presentation Worksheets

Presentation Worksheet

Idea: Diabetes

Topic: Diabetic foot care

Focus: What those with diabetes should focus on when purchasing new shoes

Purpose: To raise awareness among the lay public about the smart way to buy shoes when they or a loved one have diabetes

Audience: Lay public; 100 to 150 people

Venue: Wellness presentation in community hospital conference room; seats up to 200 people

Desired audience response: After this presentation, participants know what to consider when buying shoes for someone with diabetes.

Slant (Title): When buying new shoes, what you don't know *can* hurt you.

One-sentence description: This presentation shows how making smart choices when buying shoes can prevent serious and/or permanent foot injuries for those with diabetes.

Presentation Worksheet

Idea: _____

_____

Topic: _____

Focus: _____

Purpose: _____

Audience: _____

Venue: _____

Desired audience response: _____

Slant: _____

One-sentence description: _____

_____

Appendix B.
Kolb-It Worksheets

Kolb-It Worksheet

Idea: Stress

Snappy Title: Stress-Less Coping Strategies

CE: Soda can experiment.

RO: What was it like to imagine you'd gotten a soda can that was shaken up?

AC:

- The symptoms of stress

- The difference between "good" and "bad" stress

- Coping strategies

AE: Free-write one coping strategy from the ones listed that you will use this week to bust your stress and share this strategy with a partner.

RO: What was it like to identify and share your coping strategy?

Your Kolb-It Worksheet

Idea: _____

Snappy Title: _____

CE (Design an exercise that involves learners in their own learning.):

_____

_____

RO (Ask learners to reflect on the concrete experience.): What was

that like for you?

AC (Highlight salient theoretical points.):

_____

_____

_____

_____

AE (Allow learners to apply learning to their lives.):

_____

RO (What was that like for you?):

_____

_____

Appendix C.
Publication Worksheets

Publication Worksheet

Idea: Joy-stealing

> **Topic:** Competitive games played by nurse educators that steal joy

> **Focus:** What happens when the joy-stealer is me?

Purpose: My purpose in writing up what I learned from the participants in the joy-stealing workshop is *to inform* about how nurse educators report stealing each other's joy as well as *to move* us to examine our own behavior as joy stealers.

Readers: Academic nurses

Vehicle: *Reflections on Nursing Leadership (RNL)*

Desired Reader Response: Learn from colleagues' reflections on being joy-stealers and reflect on how they, the readers, steal other's joy.

Slant (Title): Reflective Practice

One-Sentence Description: This article will share stories from nurse educators that describe the ways they steal joy and suggest strategies for stopping the joy-stealing.

Publication Worksheet

Idea: _____

_____

Topic: _____

Focus: _____

Purpose: _____

Audience: _____

Vehicle: _____

Desired Reader Response: _____

Slant (Title): _____

One-sentence description: This article will _____

_____

Appendix D.
Timeline Worksheet

Your Timeline	
Task	**Time Frame**
1. Complete publication worksheet	(Today's Date)
2. _____	_____
3. _____	_____
4. _____	_____
5. _____	_____
6. _____	_____
7. _____	_____
8. _____	_____
9. _____	_____
10. _____	_____
	(continues)

Your Timeline

Task	Time Frame
11. _____	_____
12. _____	_____
13. _____	_____
14. _____	_____
15. _____	_____
16. _____	_____
17. _____	_____
18. _____	_____
19. _____	_____
20. _____	_____

Index